MEDICINAL
AND
AROMATIC PLANTS

(Essential Oils and Pharmaceutical Uses)

MEDICINAL AND AROMATIC PLANTS

(Essential Oils and Pharmaceutical Uses)

By

Dr. Joseph Jose

Reader

Dept. of Botany

M.G. University Centre for Research

Sacred Heart College, Thevara

Kochi, Ernakulam (Kerala)

&

Rajalakshmi, R.

Research Associate

Kerala Forest Research Institute

Peechi, Trichur (Kerala)

D P H

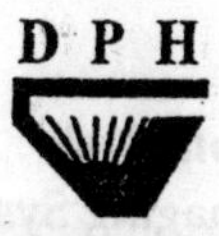

DISCOVERY PUBLISHING HOUSE

NEW DELHI-110002

First Published - 2005

Reprinted - 2015

ISBN: 978-81-7141-982-1

Medicinal and Aromatic Plants
Essential Oils & Pharmaceutical Uses

Published by:
DISCOVERY PUBLISHING HOUSE PVT. LTD.
4383/4B, Ansari Road, Darya Ganj
New Delhi-110 002 (India)
Phone: +91-11-23279245, 43596064-65
Fax: +91-11-23253475
E-mail: discoverypublishinghouse@gmail.com
sales@discoverypublishinggroup.com
web: www.discoverypublishinggroup.com

Printed at:
Infinity Imaging Systems
Delhi

Preface

In India about 20% of the 4000 tonnes of chemicals estimated to be used annually in perfumers and flavours are obtained from essential oils, which represent an important class of indigenously developed starting material for perfumery and flavour industry. Some of them are used in pharmaceutical and other industries as well. The importance of aroma chemicals and essential oils in microbiology as anti microbial agents is well established. Although more than 2000 varieties of medicinal and essential oil bearing plants are grown in our country, only a few of them have become prominent on a commercial scale.

This book is undertaken to find out the quantity of essential oil in medicinal plants with special reference to Aster family and also to identify the major components in these oils. A chemo taxonomical evaluation based on volatile oils in various plant taxa and on the range of various oil constituents suggested making use of both studies for understanding the variation and formation of taxa in nature as well as in the natural classification of plants. The medicinal aromatic and various other value added properties of Asteraceae are given in this book. However, at present many of these activities are not commonly utilised. This may be probably due to the gradual change over from herbals to synthetic drugs during the last centaury. The gradual substitution of natural aromatic oils with synthetics derived from petrochemical is very much clear. Even though a considerable amount of work has been done among the various members of Asteraceae on the chemistry of essential oils, however, they have focussed only on a few economically or commercially valuable species. The screening of a large number of lesser oil yielding plants of great medicinal importance has not been attempted so far. Only few species of the family Asteraceae has so far been phytochemically screened. The data on the chemistry of essential oils of Asteraceae too are very meagre. Considering the richness of this family in the vegetation of India, it has been thought that a systematic work with regard to its essential oil constituents and their significance may lead to a better understanding of these plants because most of the plants of Asteraceae are used in folk medicines or grand mother's remedy for common diseases.

The available information concerning the drugs and medicinal plants of India is scattered through a number of books and periodicals in various languages, as well as official documents, which have only had a very limited circulation. The authors of this book how presented to the public have endeavored to collect and verify this information, and supplement it where deficient by original investigation especially directed towards the elucidation of the chemical composition and physiological action of the plants and drugs.

Nature has been the biggest architect of heterogeneous chemical especially in case of plant kingdom where they have been used to ward off unwanted insects, pests, rodents, predators or to deferred against various diseases, herbivory or even to attract pollinators. The natural purpose of the synthesis and accumulation of terpenoids in the plant kingdom still possess a considerable question mark to phytochemists. They have some role in plant growth regulation, in pollination biology, in various interactions with other plants, animals or insects, in defence against diseases and in other attacks. However, the studies on the chemical defensive mechanism of terpenoids are still at an early stage. Hence, it is high time to collect sufficient data and to emphasis duly the ecological role of terpenoids as primarily defensive agents against over grazing. This topic therefore, offers ample scope for future research programmers and pharmaceutical industries as well.

Introduction

More than 2000 varieties of medicinal and essential oil bearing plants are grown in our country, only a few of them have become prominent on a commercial scale. Medicinal plants have curative properties due to the presence of various complex chemical substances of different compounds which are found as secondary metabolites in one or more parts of the plants. The medicinal value of the drug plants is due to the presence of these specific chemical substances present in them, which when consumed in small doses, produces physiological action in the human body. Some of these important compounds include alkaloids, glucosides, resins, gums, mucilage, tannins, essential oils, compounds of hydrogen, oxygen, and nitrogen etc. and these compounds are generally present in the roots, stems, leaves, barks and seeds.

The use of plants as source of medicine dates backs to about 4000 to 5000 B. C. The Chinese were to pioneers in using plants as valuable source of medicine. Drug plants had been extensively described by Aristotle and Theophrastus, early in 77 BC. In early times plants were studied mainly from the standpoint of their food and medicinal value.

Human beings have been dependent on higher plants for their health care needs since the very beginning of human civilization. In addition to food, clothing and shelter, the green plants have provided all the medicinal to man and its domestic animals for thousands of year. Initially the plants were the main part of folk medicine practiced by the ancient man in different parts of the world which include, India, China, Middle East, Africa and South America. The folk medicine in various countries gave rise to traditional system of medicine. Some of the most important system still practiced in the third world countries especially Yunani practiced in India, Pakistan, Afghanistan, Bangladesh and the Middle East. Ayurveda and Siddha practiced in India, Nepal, Bangladesh and Sri Lanka and the Chinese system of medicine employed in China and other far Eastern Countries derive more than 80% of therapeutic agents from plants.

From folk medicine and traditional system of Medicine, Medicinal plants were adopted into modern system of Medicine after they have been found effective drugs through chemical and pharmaceutical screening. In the initial stages of development of modern medicine, plants and plant products formed important part of pharmacopoeia. However because of significant development in synthetic drug chemistry and antibiotics there was certain amount of decline in the use of plants in modern medicine and at one time one would have thought that alternately chemists will be able to synthesis all the active constituents of plants which are required by the modern medicine. In India, medicinal plants have made a good, contribution to the development of ancient Indian Materia Medica . One of the earliest tretiser on Indian medicine, the Charak Samhitha (1000BC), records the use of over 340 drugs of vegetable origin. Most of these continue to be gathered from wild plants to meet the demand of the medicinal profession. Thus, despite the rich heritage of knowledge on the use of plant drugs, little attention had been paid to grow them as field crops in the country till the latter part of the nineteenth century.

Traditional herbal medicine is becoming popular in India for the treatment of several diseases. In general the use of the herbal drugs is recognized by the people of India as being safer than the modern allopathic ones. In India numerous plants are used to treat various diseases in ethanomedical practices in remote villages and tribal pockets. Many plants seen around us are used as grand mothers remedy for common chills, fever and cold.

India is immensely blessed with much biological and cultural heritage. The flora, fauna and other natural resource systems in this country are a good source of potential raw materials for bioindustrial development. This natural resource base is complemented with an equally rich and diverse cultural heritage and traditional knowledge systems. The medicinal plant wealth, the strong and time tested traditional medicare systems like Ayurveda and the human resource base are the strengths of India. The Ayurveda and other green health traditions of India have started gaining high appreciation and acceptance in the industrialized countries. Ayurveda thus offers India tremendous scope not only for earning foreign exchange but also for production of a wide range of herbal drugs and pharmaceuticals through scientific validation and standardization techniques.

Herbal Technology and Information Technology would be the two challenging enterprises, which India could adopt to meet its immediate economic growth and social development. The biological resources, particularly medicinal plant resources and the associated indigenous knowledge, innovations, traditions and practices are an important asset of our country, which could be judiciously exploited through appropriate scientific and technological inputs. Herbal Technology alone can perhaps help India to convert its biological capital to economic wealth. Such enterprises, if meticulously planned and executed, could help generate more opportunities for employment and income in rural as well as urban sectors. In order to achieve sustainable economic growth India should now take up a comprehensive action-oriented research and development programme in bioprospecting of medicinal plant resources of the country. Building up necessary scientific infrastructure and capability in advanced biotechnologies like high-through put chemical screening, DNA fingerprinting, gene cloning, transgenics, instrumentation and enzyme technologies are the prerequisites to undertake chemical and gene prospecting of medicinal plants in India. Conservation and cultivation of wild medicinal plants are also required to be undertaken simultaneously to ensure the continued supply of quality raw materials

Many herbal remedies individually or in combination with formulation such as leaf powder, pastes, decoction, infusion, pills etc. have been recommended in various medical treatises for different ointment. Our locality is abundant of rich sources of medicinal plants. Many families are rich source of medicinal plants.

Asteraceae, Lamiaceae, and Meliaceae are some. There are many studies about medicinal plants and these studies consisted to research the usefulness of many taxa in traditional medicine and pharmacopy and included the preparation of the medicines and their indications.

This book gives information to find out the quantity of essential oil in medicinal plants of Aster family and also to identify the major components in these oils. A chemo taxonomical evaluation based on volatile oils in various plant taxa and on the range of various oil constituents suggested making use of both studies for understanding the variation and formation of taxa in nature as well as in the natural classification of plants.

Contents

Preface

Introduction

1. Terpenoids **1-9**

2. Characterisation of Essential Oils in Aster Family **10-27**

3. Chemical Composition of the Essential Oil of Asteraceae **28-410**

Achillea Abrotanoides 28-29

Achillea biebersteinii (Turkey) 1 30-31

Achillea biebersteinii (Turkey) 2 32-34

Achillea collina 35

Achillea ligustica flower (Greece) 36-37

Achillea ligustica leaf (Greece) 38-39

Achillea wilhelmsii (Egypt) 40-42

Achillea wilhelmsii (Turkey) 43-44

Achillea wilnelmsii (Egypt) 45-47

Yarrow (Iran) 48-49

Yarrow 50-51

Yarrow (France) 52-53

Ageratum houstonianum (India) 54-56

Ambrosia artemisiafolia 57-58

Shanqui 59-60
Annual wormwood (Vietnam) 1 b 61-62
Roman chamomile (India) 63-65
Roman chamomiie (Italy) 1 66-67
Roman chamomile (Italy) 3 68
Roman chamomiie (Italy) 2 (headspace) 69
Roman chamomile (Italy) 5 70
Roman chamomile (Italy) 4 71
Roman chamomile (Egypt) 72
Roman chamomile (England) 73
Roman chamomile (Japan) 74-75
Artemisia abaensis (China) 76-77
Artemisia abrotanum (Italy) 78-80
Wormwood (Mugwort) (India) 81
Wormwood (Mugwort) (Spain) 82-83
Wormwood (Mugwort) 84-85
Wormwood (Mugwort), headspace 86
Wormwood (Mugwort) (Germany) 87-88
Wormwood (Mugwort) (U.S.A.) 1 89-90
Wormwood (Mugwort) (Italy) 1 91-92
Wormwood (Mugwort) (U.S.A.) 2 93-94
Wormwood (Mugwort) (U.S.A.) 3 95
Wormwood (Mugwort) (Italy) 2 96-98
Wormwood (Mugwort) (U.S.A.) 4 99-100
Wormwood (Mugwort) (U.S.A.) 5 101-102
Lanyana (Oregon-USA) 103
Lanyana (South Africa) 104
Lanyana (Zimbabwe) 105
Artemisia afra Willd. (Kenia) 106-107
Artemisia aksaiensis (China) 108-109
Artemisia alba (Belgium) 110-111
Artemisia alba (Italy) 112-114
Artemisia anethifoiia (China) 115

Artemisia anethoides (China)	116
Annual wormwood (USA, Oregon)	117
Annual wormwood (India)	118
Annual wormwood 2	119
Annual wormwood 1	120
Annual wormwood, leaf (U.S.A.,Indiana)1	121-122
Annual wormwood, leaf (U.S.A., Indiana) 2	123-124
Annual wormwood, flower (U.S.A., Indiana)	125-126
Annual wormwood (Mongolia)	127
Annual wormwood (China) 1	128-129
Annual wormwood (Yugoslavia)	130-131
Annual wormwood (France)	132-133
Annual wormwood (China) 2a	134-135
Annual wormwood (China) 2b	136-137
Annual wormwood (Vietnam)1a	138-139
Annual wormwood (Hungary)	140
Annual wormwood (Italy)	141-143
Artemisia arborescens (U.S.A.)	144-145
Artemisia argentea (Madeira)	146-147
Arternisia atrovirens (China)	148-149
Artesimia campestris (Italy) 2	150-152
Artemisia chamaemelifolia (Italy)	153-155
Artemisia desertorum (China)	156
Tarragon (USA) 1	157-158
Tarragon (USA) 2	159-160
Tarragon (USA) 3	161-162
Tarragon (USA) 4	163-164
Estragon	165
Tarragon (France) 1	166
Tarragon (France) 2	167
Tarragon (Italy)	168
Tarragon	169-170
Tarragon (Cuba)	171-172

Artemisia genipi (Italy)	173-175
Artemisia glacialis (Italy)	176-178
Artemisia gmelini (Himalaya)	179-180
Armoise (Morocco)	181-182
Artemisia indica (China)	183
Artemisia judaica (Israel) 1	184-186
Artemisia Judaica (Egypt) 1	187-188
Artemisia judaica (Egypt) 2	189-190
Artemisia judaica (Israel) 2	191-193
Artemisia kawakamii (China)	194
Arteinisia macrocephaia (China)	195
Artemisia maritima (Himalaya)	196
Artemisia molinieri	197-198
Artemisia monosperma	199-200
Artemisia moorcroftiana	201-203
Artemisia nilagirica (vulgaris) (India) 2	204-205
Artemisia nilagirica (vulgaris) (India) 1	206-207
Artemisia occidentalis-sichaunensis (China)	208-209
Davana 1	210
Davana (India) 1	211-212
Davana (India) 2	213-214
Artemisia persica (India)	215-216
Artemisia petrosa (Italy)	217-216
Wormwood Roman, headspace	220
Wormwood Roman	221-222
Artemisia princeps (China)	223-224
Artemisia pubescens (China)	225
Artemisia roburghiana (Himalaya)	226-227
Artemisia scoparia (India)	228
Artemisia speciosa (China)	229
Artemisia subulata (China)	230
Artemisia umbelliformis (Italy)	231-233
Artemisia valiesiaca (Italy)	234-236

Artemisia verlotiorum (Italy)	237-239
Artemisia vestita (India)	240-241
Armoise flower	242-244
Artemisia vulgaris (Italy)	245-247
Artemisia Waltonii (China)	248
Baccharis genistelloides	249-250
Blumea brevipes	251-253
Blumea lanceolaria	254
Muhuhu	255
Marigoid pot 1	256-258
Marigold pot 2	259-260
Chamomile (Argentina)	261
Chamomile (Hungary)	262
Chamomile (Brazil)	263
Chamomile (Germany) 1	264-265
Chainomile (Germany) 2, Living Flower	266-267
Carlina acauiis root	268
Chariioinile (Bulgaria)	269
Chamomile (Egypt)	270
Chamomile (Italy) 1	271
Chamomile (Italy) 2	272-273
Chamomile, wild (Morocco)	274-275
Balsamite	276-277
Conyza pinnata (Zimbabwe)	278
Conyza sumatrensis	279
Coreopsis barteri leaf (Cameroon)	280-281
Coreopsis grandiflora leaf (Cameroon)	282-283
Dendranthema vestitum flower absolute (China)	284-285
Egietes viscosa (flower heads)	286-287
Erigeron Canadensis	288-289
Eupatorium argentinum leaf	290-291
Eupatorium arnottianum leaf	292-293
Eupatorium hecatanthum leaf	294-295

Eupatorium maximilianii	296-297
Eupatorium stoechadosmum	298
Eupatorium subhastatum leaf	299-300
Grinciela robusta	301
Grindeia squarrosa	302
Helichrysum hypnoides (Madagascar)	303
Helichrysum odoratissimum	304
Helichrysum bracteiferum (Madagascar)	305
Heterotheca inuloides leaf (Mexico)	306-307
Ichtyothere terminalis (Brazil)	308-309
Inula viscosa (Turkey)	310-312
Pectis prostrata leaf	313-314
Psiadia lithospermifolia	315
Psiadia viscosa	316-317
Pteronia incana 1	318
Pteronia incana 2	319-320
Santolina chamaecyparissus (France) 1	321-322
Santolina chamaecyparissus (France) 2	323-325
Pectis elongata	326-327
Santolina chamaecyparissus (France) 3	328-329
Santolina chamaecyparissus (Egypt)	330-332
Santolina neapolitana (Italy)	333-334
Santolina pectina	335-336
Santolina canescens	337-338
Santolina rosmarinifolia	339-340
Santolina semidentata	341-342
Senecio	343-344
Sphaeranthus cyathuloides (Kenya)	345
Sphaeranthus suaveolens (Egypt)	346-347
Tagetes argentina 1 (Argentina)	348
Tagetes argentina 2 (Argentina)	349
Tagetes argentina 3 (Argentina)	350
Tagetes filifolia (Argentina) 1	351

Tagetes filifolia (Argentina) 2	352
Tagetes laxa (Argentina)	353
Tagetes lemmonii	354
Tagetes lucida (Hungary)	355
Tagetes (Argentina) 1	356
Tagetes (India) 1	357
Tagetes (India) 2	358
Tagetes (USA) 1	359
Tagetes 1	360
Tagetes 2	361-363
Tagetes (India) 5	364
Tagetes (India) 4	365
Tagetes (Argentina) 2a	366
Tagetes (Argentina) 2b	367
Tagetes (India) 3	368
Tagetes (USA) 2	369-370
Tagetes 3a (leaf)	371
Tagetes 3b (flower)	372
Tagetes (Rwanda)	373-374
Tagetes (France)	375-376
Tagetes minuta (Hungary)	377
Tagetes (Turkey)	378-379
Tagetes patula (Hungary)	380
Tagetes riojana (Argentina)	381
Tagetes tenuifolia (Hungary)	382
Tagetes terniflora (Argentina)	383
Tanacetum parthenium (Belgium)	384-385
Tanacetum parthenium (The Netherlands)	386-387
Tansy (Belgium)	388-389
Tansy flowers (Canada)	390-391
Tansy stems & sheets (Canada)	392-393
Tithonia diversifolia	394-395
Vanillosmopsis arborea leaf	396

Vanillosmopsis arborea bark	397
Vassaoura (Uruguay)	398-399
Vassoura (Brazil) 1	400
Vassoura (Brazil) 2	401-402
Vassoura (Brazil) 3	403-407
Wedelia paludosa (Brazil) 1	408-409
Wedelia paludosa (Brazil) 2	410
References	*411*
Glossary of Medical Terms	*415*

1

Terpenoids

An enormous range of plant substances are covered by the word 'terpenoid' a term which is used to indicate that all such substances have a common biosynthetic origin. Terpenoids range from the essential oil components, the volatile mono and sesquiterpenes, through the less volatile diterpenes to the non-volatile triterpens and sterols. Each of these various classes of terpenoids are of significance in plant growth, metabolism or ecology. Chemically terpenoids are generally lipid soluble and are located in the cytoplasm of the plant cell. A considerable number of quite different functions have been ascribed to plant terpenoids. Their growth regulating properties are very well documented; two of the major classes of growth regulators are the sesquiterpenoid abscisins and the diterpenoid based gibberellins. Less is generally known of the role of terpenoids in the more subtle interactions between plants and animals as agents of communication and defence among insects, but this is now an area of active research. Many studies have demonstrated that terpenoids display a wide range of pharmacological activities. Some of these compounds have been identified the active principles of crude drugs used in folk medicines.

Chemically terpenoids are usually unsaturated hydrocarbons, with varying degree of oxygenation in the substituent groups (alcohol, aldehyde, lactone etc.) attached to the basic skeleton. The terpenoids are known to have as diverse functions as their chemical structures. They have specific role in many of the plant-animal, plant-plant and plant-micro organism interactions as phytoalexins, insect antifeedants, defence agents, pheromones, allelochemicals, signal molecules and so on. Some are highly toxic to animal systems while others have the ability to interfere hormonally with insect metamorphosis and with animal growth and reproduction.

Terpenoids are generally lipid soluble and are located in the cytoplasm of the plant cell. Two classes of terpene, mono and sesquiterpenes differ in their boiling point range (monoterpenes b.p 140-180°, sesquiterpenes b.p>200°) simple monoterpenes are wide spread and tend to occur as components of the majority of essential oils. True sesquiterpenes accompany monoterpenes in plant essential oils, although because of their higher molecular weight, they are in the less volatile fraction. The sesquisterpene lactones, are lipophilic substances secreted in leaf trichomes, waxes, and in latexes. Some of the sweet smelling terpenoids are attractants to insects for oviposition on the one hand and ovicidal on the other hand. Some terpenoids attract the scavengers who feed on plant eating insects. Pinene which is present in many plants show high repellent activity against certain insects while germacrene-D, a sesquiterpene hydrocarbon is reported to be a male sex stimulant for certain cockroaches. Limonene and alpha-pinene has the property to mimic, alarm or alter pheromones of certain termites. The chemical components such as camphene, cineole, eugenol, geraniol, limonene, linalool, beta-phellandrene and alpha-pinene have been reported for their insecticidal and ovicidal actions.

Very little is known regarding the role of diterpenoids and triterpenoids. Most of the diterpenes are notable for their irritant and co-carcinogenic properties. Various ecological functions of the diterpenes in the plant kingdom such as defence against herbivory, hormonal interference in insects, antifeedant activity, phytoallexin defense and antifungal defense are reported.

Chemical Ecology of Terpenoids in Asteraceae

The various species coming under the family Asteraceae show different levels of chemical adaptations to their environment.

Many members of this family are aromatic and sesquiterpenic lactones, usually non-volatile, called bitter principles or resins occurs frequently and these should be a clear function for their secondary metabolites in the well being of these plants in their surrounding environment.

Monoterpenes also occur in Asteraceae plants. Their ecological role as pollinator attraction is clearly proved. These terpenens also accumulate in quantity in leaves and stems. Some compounds are regularly, found together in leaf oils, especially alpha and beta-pinene, limonene, alpha-phellandrene and myrcene. Flower and seed oils tend to have more specialized monoterpenes present. Most of these components have a defensive role against herbivory. They are either toxic or deterrent to a range of herbivory and represent a real barrier to feeding. Limonene possesses strong feeding inhibitory activity. Terpenen-4-ol and alpha-terpineol often exert great anti feedant effect by contact action .The production of these terpenoids in the leafy shoot region protects plant tissues from herbivory and the concentration of these components increases in response to herbivory. Monoterpenes are probably toxic to most insects, not adapted to them. They are also toxic to microorganisms and have allelopathic effects on plant tissues. The species of *Ageratum* are found to be allelopathic to many of the surrounding under shrubs. The monoterpenes present in the leaves of such plants may be released into the environment and exert an allelopathic influence on other plant species preventing their growth.

The sesquiterpenes accompany monoterpenes in plant essential oils, although because of their molecular weight, they are in the less volatile fraction. Sesquiterpenes have a common occurrence in the essential oil of Asteraceae. Two derived sesquiterpenoids abscisic acid and xanthinin deserve special mention. Abscisic acid is best known as the principal hormone controlling dormancy in seeds of herbaceous plants and in buds of woody plant. Xanthinin, which occurs in cocklebur, *Xanthium pennsylvanicum* has a well-defined role in plant physiology as an auxin antagonist.

The biological activities associated with sesquiterpenes, are many and varied, from plant growth regulation (abscissic acid) to interference with insect metamorphosis. Some sesquiterpenes protect plants from insect attack because of their antimicrobial properties. This appears to be true of caryophyllene and caryophyllene epoxide, which are repellent to the leaf cutting ants *Attacephalotes* and *Acromyrmex octopinosus.* Caryophyllene is present in almost all investigated species. Caryophyllene epoxide in particular occurs in the leaf of *Melampodium divaricatum* and protects the plant from ant cutting activities. The ants reject the leaves because the epoxide damges the fungus, upon which they depend for their food.

The important class of sequiterpenes, sesquiterpene lactons, which have a wide distribution in the family Asteraceae. This sequiterpene lactons of which some 5000 are now known, are lipophilic substances secreted in leaf trichomes, waxes and in latexes. These also have an important role in plants of Asteraceae as chemical defence agents. They are often present in high concentration and relatively complex mixtures of different structures are found in many species. Usually bitter tasting, they are obviously deterrent to many kinds of herbivore, including man himself. Their effects on insects are very damaging and they are also poisonous to livestock. Other properties possessed by these sesquiterpene lactones include their pungent taste and their ability to act as allergens. The sesquiterpene lactones likewise have a wide range of demonstrated biological activities, as cytotoxic compounds, vertebrate poisons insect feeding deterrents, schistosomicidal substances, and allergenic agents.

There is much indirect evidence that sesquiterpene lactones cause insect herbivores to avoid plants containing them because of their antifeedant growth inhibitory or toxic effects. However, ecological data confirming the defensive role of these lactones in the plants where they occur are still relatively limited. The lactones caused severe growth inhibition and antifeedant activity against six lepidopterous larvae, in some *Vernonia* species *(V.glanca* and *V. gigantea)*. One of the noted features of various aromatic species is that, they show anti herbivory and this may be due to the terpene present in the leafy and shoot portions. Herbivorous animals like deer and rabbit are not often eating some *Vernonia* species (*V.glanca* and *V. gigantea*). Species of *Eupatorium* are very resistant to many diseases. They are not even effected by many bacterial, viral and fungal diseases. The essential oil constituent present in *Chromolaena odorata* exhibited activity against Escherichia coli, Pseudomonas aeruginosa and Klebsiella pneumoniae. *Ageratum* oil was inhibitory to some fungi. There are many reports about the protective role of diterpenes against herbivory in florets of the Sunflower, *Helianthus annuus*. This diterpenes are both growths inhibitory and larvicidal to the sunflower moth Homeosoma.

Aromatic Plants

Aromatic plants possess odorous volatile substances, which occur as essential oil, gum exudates, balsam and oleoresin in one or more parts, namely root, wood, bark, stem, foliage, flower and fruit. The characteristic aroma is due to a variety of complex chemical compounds. The term essential oil is concomitant to fragrance or perfumes because these fragrances are oily in nature and they represent the essence or the active constituents of the plants. They are called volatile or ethereal oils as they evaporate when exposed to air at ordinary temperatures. Essential oils are highly concentrated, low volume, high value products.

Essential Oils

The essential oils comprise the volatile steam – distillable fraction responsible for the characteristic scent, odour or smell found in many plants. They are commercially important as the basis of natural perfumes, and also of spices and flavouring in the food industry. The term 'essential oil' is open to wide interpretation and may include products obtained by traditional methods of distillation, and those obtained by very selective solvent extraction or medicinal expression. Plant families particularly rich in essential oils include the Asteraceae, Labiatae, Myrtaceae, Rosaceae, Rutaceae, and Umbelliferae. Essential oils sometimes occur in special glandular cells on the leaf surface whilst carotenoids are especially associated with chloroplasts in the leaf and with chromoplasts in the petal.

Essential oils, nevertheless, differ from fixed oils. The former can be distilled from their natural sources, do not consist of glyceryl esters of fatty acids thereby not having a permanent oily spot on paper and are unsaponifiable with alkalies. Essential oils have several common physical properties like characteristic fragrances and high refractive indices. They are mostly optically active and immiscible with water but sufficiently soluble to impact their characteristic fragrance to water. Factually, the aromatic waters are dependable on this slight solubility. Essential oils are however soluble in ether, alcohol and organic solvents.

Essential oils are colourless or lightly coloured and free flowing when they are fresh. On long storage they become darker in colour and highly viscous due to oxidation and resinification. To prevent this, they are stored in a cool and dry place in tightly stoppered amber glass bottles. Exclusion of air by completely filling the containers with oil prolongs its storage life. This deterioration in quality of the oil is attributed to a number of chemical reaction such as oxidation, resinification, polymerization, hydrolysis of esters and interaction of functional group.

Particularly all volatile oils have complex mixtures of chemicals varying widely in chemical composition and having many organic compounds (oxides, esters, aldehydes, ketones, ethers, alcohols and hydrocarbons). Only a few possess a single component in a high percentage viz. santalol in sandal wood oil, citral in lemongrass oil and eugenol in cinnamon oil. The diverse type of organic compounds are, however, separated by various techniques, a few are given below:

1. Fractional distillation;
2. Fractional crystallization from poor solvents;
3. Removal by chemical action. Free acidic group is removed from the oil by Na_2CO_3; basic compounds are removed with HCl, phenols with NaOH and aldehydes with $NaHSO_3$ and so forth.

Processes like steam-distillation, hydro-diffusion, hydro-distillation, enfleurage, maceration, expression and solvent extraction are available. Application of these processes either singly or in combination, depends upon the nature of the material and of the essential oil or absolute intended to be recovered. A brief resume of these is given here.

Distillation

The three systems are (i) hydro-distillation (ii) hydro-steam distillation and (iii) steam distillation.

In all these processes, it is intensity of steam that differs to carry the volatile odouriferous oil along with its vapours and condensed to liquefy the oil and steam vapours. To get maximum extraction, flowers and leaves by virtue of their having desired thinness of the cell walls are not comminuted. Others are subjected to comminution.

(i) The hydro-distillation system though being the oldest is still being practiced. The plant material is in direct contact with boiling water in a crude metallic distillation outfit.

(ii) The hydro-steam distillation system is employed where the perfumery material is vulnerable to direct steam. Consequently, the material is supported on a perforated grid or screen inserted at some distance above the bottom of the still. The lower part of the still contains water up to a level just below the grid. Pressure steam is passed. With each new batch, the water at the bottom of the still is changed.

(iii) In the steam-distillation system, live steam at 5 +/- 2-kgs/sq. cm. is injected through steam coils below the charge and the pressure within the distillation vessel is controlled according to the nature of the material being distilled. This method is not applicable to delicate flowers, however, is better than the above methods. It gives better, cheaper and quicker yield.

Rectification of distillates is effected by fractional hydro-distillation at reduced pressure for improving their colour. Bad odours and impurities are removed in the foreruns during rectification.

As reported elsewhere, the major odouriferous constituents of most of the essential oils are oxygenated compounds like alcohols, aldehydes, esters, ethers, ketones, lactones, phenols and phenol ethers. Terpenes and sequiterpenes are usually present along with these compounds and their separation is beneficial. This is effected through fractional distillation in vaccum, alternatively, alternatively by solvent extraction. Usually the terpeneless oil is extracted with dilute alcohol or similar solvents to remove waxes and sesquiterpenes. Frequently advantages is taken of differential solubility of the oil components in two solvents partially soluble in each other, flowering the oil counter current to the solvent mixture. Example, pentane and dilute methanol mixture. Pentane dissolves the terpenes and methanol the above described oxygenated.

The aforesaid methods are long, tardy and require the skill to avoid thermal or hydrolytic damage to the delicate components. Though still practiced by medium range perfumers, these have been substituted by recent chromatographic systems of gas chromatography, gas-liquid chromotography, and high performance liquid chromatography.

The Gas Chromatographic (GC) methods are proved to be effective when unknown oil samples are subjected to this technique. The versatility of the gas chromatographic methods provides information not only about the number of constituents in the sample but the constituents are quantified with high precision even when microgram levels of samples are available. This method also provides easy and effective detection of foreign constituents in the essential oil.

Gas Liquid Chromatography (GLC) is an excellent tool for the separation, characterisation and quantitative estimation of volatile components of essential oils. Separation of components from the oil that formerly took days by classical methods can now be accomplished within minutes. It has the added advantage of requiring very small quantity of the sample, say a microgram.

A recently developed technique regarding the analysis of total essential oil is GC-MS. This technique is now increasingly used for the analysis of essential oils. GC as it is already discussed, is a tool for separating the volatile components while analysis depends upon retention characteristics under standard conditions. The mass spectrometer can be used as a detector for a gas chromatograph in which case, the high degree of specificity of the mass spectrum is an aid to the identification of the sample. The large number of spectra obtained in a short time from the GC – MS technique and the routine nature of the data obtained, makes the computer a very useful accessory to the GC-MS unit. With the help of GC-MS technique it has now been possible to analyse directly the fragrances of natural as well as artificial material without the use of heat or solvents directly by the use of head space analysis. A GC-MS machine, which has computerized library search discs, can be regarded as the best single tool for essential oil analysis.

Finally, a mention may also be made of High Pressure Liquid Chromatography (HPLC), which can also be useful for separation, identification and estimation of solids, and high boiling liquids, which are otherwise very difficult to resolve, by GLC.

2

Characterisation of Essential Oils in Aster Family

The Asteraceae family is one of the most numerous within the Phanerogames. This dicotyledonous family is widely distributed and constitutes about 10% of the entire population of flowering plants. The members of this family show a remarkable diversity in habit. Asteraceae has been thought to be at or very near the peak of dicot evolution. This family is readily distinguishable from all other families by the flowers aggregated together in head or capitulam. The number of florets in a head varies enormously from several thousands as in huge heads of some sunflowers, to a single flower, as in *Echinops*, where, the single flowered head is however, generally associated in secondary heads. Florets of a head is bisexual or unisexual (monecious or dioecious) or the outer (ray florets) female or asexual. Many members of the family are of economic or medicinal value from the presence of ethereal and fatty oils, resins and bitter principles. Many indigenous plants are used as grandmother's remedy for common colds, chills and fever. Asteraceae are chemically characterised by synthesis and accumulation of many classes of natural products. Complex antibiotic preparations are also obtained from some members of Asteraceae Insecticides, oils, dyes, and edible products are prepared from some members.

Plant Materials

The whole plant body can be collected for the extraction of essential oils, to get maximum yield of oil. The collection should be made during the period May – December, peak flowering season for the members of Asteraceae, since essential oil production in many members of the family is at the highest level during florescence stage. Moreover, the plant materials should collect during early afternoon because maximum content of volatile oil occur at that period. The plant materials collected should clean and shade dried at room temperature, because shade drying reduces the weight of the herb to 1/3 of the fresh weight and maximizes the oil yield with out affecting the quality of the essential oil.

Isolation of Essential Oil

Separation of the volatile oils from the dried flaked and powdered plant tissue can be conducted by hydro distillation in a Clevenger apparatus for 4 to 5 hours, as prolonged extraction normally increases the yield. Extraction should be carried out at ambient temperature to necessitate economy. The percentage of essential oils is calculated on a dry weight basis to avoid faulty estimation that may arise due to the different water content of the tissue analysed each time. The isolated oil is then dried over anhydrous sodium sulphate and stored at 4 to 6° C.

Qualitative Analysis

Qualitative estimation of the essential oils can be done by capillary Gas chromatography. For each plant, GC analysis can performed by using a Chemito Gas Chromatograph (model CHEMITO 8510) equipped with a flame ionization detector (FID). The capillary GC can be carried out on 5% SE – 30 packed column with the following dimensions mesh size – 80/100; length – 8 feet; diameter – 1/8 inch. Nitrogen should use as carrier gas at '10 psi (inlet pressure) with a flow rate of 30 ml/minute. Temperature programming is performed from 80° C to 230° C at the rate of 6° C/minute. Major components are identified by retention time (RT) analysis and peak enrichment by co-injection with authentic standards. Relative retention times of these reference standards are obtained by taking gas chromatograms of their mixtures in similar conditions.

1. *Ageratum conizoides* Linn- The plant is an erect herb, annual, 30-60cm, hispidly hairy, leaves petioled, ovate crenate, heads small in dense terminal corymbs, homogamous flowers blue or white.

Value Added Property

• In cuts and sores and as an external application in ague	Leaves
• In vitiated conditions of kapha and vata, dyspepsia, anorexia purulent ophthalmia, renal and vesical calculi and pharyngopathy	Roots
• In haemorrhoids, wounds sores and boils	Leaves
• As a lotion for eyes and for treating fresh cuts and wounds	Leaf juice
• Anti inflammatory and analgesic	Roots
• In cephagia, dyspnea, fever and enteralgia	Plant
• For antispasmodic, anti asthmatic, haemostic and insecticidal properties	Crude extract
• In intestinal disorders and inflammatory stomach	Stem and leaf
• Antibacterial and Antifungal	Oil

Major Essential Oil Components

- Unidentified – 64.2%, beta-Elemene – 3.6%, beta-Bisabolene – 2.5%, beta-Caryophyllene – 2.4%, alpha-Pinene – 0.85%, beta-Phellandrene – 0.61%
- 31.10%-Precocene II, 29.00%-Precocene I, 2.50%-Camphene, 2.30%-beta-Farnesene, 2.00%-beta-Selinene, 2.00%-beta-Cubebene,1.90%-alpha-Terpinene,1.20%-Bornyl acetate,1.00%-beta-Elemene,0.90%-Myrcene,0.50%-Caryophyllene oxide, 0.40%-alpha-Pinene,0.40%-beta-Pinene,0.40%-alpha-Cubebene,0.40%-6-Vinyl demethoxyageratochromene, 0.30%-Borneol, 0.20%-Farnesol (unknown isomer),0.10%-beta-Caryophyllene
- 38.50%-Precocene I, 20.05%-beta-Caryophyllene, 17.65%-Precocene II, 5.75%-alpha-Farnesene, 1.25%-Bicyclo

[3.2.1]oct-2-ene, 3-methyl-4-methylene, 1.10%-Germacrene D, 0.85%-Farnesene (unknown isomer), 0.65%-beta-Cubebene, 0.55%-gamma-Cadinene, 0.55%-Germacrene (unknown isomer), 0.45%-Terpinen-4-yl acetate, 0.35%-beta-Elemene, 0.35%-alpha-Elemene, 0.30%-alpha-Cubebene, 0.25%-gamma-Elemene, 0.10%-Caryophyllene oxide, 0-01%-alpha-Copaene, 0.01%-beta-Bourbonene

- .90%-beta-Farnesene, 1.85%-Sesquiterpene hydrocarbons (unknown),1.35%-delta-Cadinene,48.80%-Precocene I, 18.95%-beta-Caryophyllene,10.80%-PrecoceneII, 5.25%-alpha-Farnesene, 4.35%-beta-Farnesene, 2.05%-alpha-Humulene,1.25%-Bicyclogermacrene, 0.75%-GermacreneD, 0.70%-Sesquiterpene hydrocarbons (unknown), 0.60%-Terpinen-4-yl acetate, 0.55%-delta-Cadinene, 0.50%-beta-Cubebene, 0-45%-Caryophyllene oxide, 0.45% ~ Farnesene (unknown isomer), 0.40%-gamma-Elemene, 0.35%-gamma-Cadinene,0.35%-beta-Elemene,0.35%-alpha-Elemene,0.15%-Germacrene (unknown isomer),0.01%-alpha-Copaene,0.01%-alpha-Cubebene,0.01%-beta-Bourbonene
- 45.05%-PrecoceneI, 19.60%-beta-Caryophyllene,10.00%-Precocene II, 6.45%-beta-Farnesene,3.50%-alpha-Farnesene, 3.15%-alpha-Humulene,2.15%-Germacrene D, 1.95%-Bicyclogermacrene,1.25%-delta-Cadinene, 1.05%-Farnesene (unknown isomer), 0.85%-beta-Cubebene, 0.65%-gamma-Cadinene, 0.55%-Terpinen-4-yl acetate, 0.55%-Sesquiterpene hydrocarbons (unknown), 0.35%-beta-Elemene, 0.30%-alpha-Elemene, 0.25%-alpha-Cubebene, 0.20%-Germacrene (unknown isomer),0.10%-gamma-Elemene, 0.05%-alpha-Copaene, 0.05%-Caryophyllene oxide, 0.01%-beta Bourbonene
- 34.90%-Precocene II, 30.30%-Precocene I,14.30%-beta-Caryophyllene, 2.30%-gamma-Cadinene,1.60%-6-Vinyl-7-methoxy-2, 2-dimethylchromene,1.10%-beta-Bisabolene, 0.80%-alpha-Phellandrene,0.40%-Bornyl acetate, 0.30%-delta-Cadinene,0.10%-gamma-Terpinene, 0.10%-alpha-Muurolene,0.10%-alpha-Copaene,0.05%-alpha-Pinene,0.05%-Camphene, 0.05%-Sabinene 0.05%-beta-

Pinene,0.05%-Limonene, 0.05%-alpha-Cubebene, 0.05%-(Z)-beta-Farnesene, 0.05%-Bornyl formate

- 36.90%-Precocene II, 26.60%-Precocene I,17.00%-beta-Caryophyllene, 2.10%-beta-Bisabolene,1.70%-alpha-Farnesene, 1.30%-gamma-Muurolene,0.40%-alpha-Cubebene, 0.20%-alpha-Copaene,0.10%-Bornyl acetate, 0.10%-Demethoxyencecalin,0.05%-alpha-Bergamotene, 0.05%-6-Vinyl-7-metnoxy-2,2-dimethylchromene
- 60.13%-Precocene II, 21.25%-Precocene I,8.34%-beta-Caryophyllene, 1.07%-beta-Farnesene,0.93%-Coumarin, 0.75%-Camphene,0.74%-Bornyl acetate, 0.72%-3-Hexenol-1M,0.69%-gamma-Elemene, 0.47%-beta-Cubebene
- 80.29%-Precocene I, 7.04%-beta-Caryophyllene, 2.71%-alpha-Pinene,0.77%-GermacreneD,0.68%-beta-Sesquiphellandrene,0.67%-gamma-Elemene, 0.52%-beta-Phellandrene,0.41%-Camphene,0.32%-(Z)-beta-Farnesene,0.30%-delta-Cadinene, 0.29%-(E)-Nerolidol,0.28%-Bornyl acetate, 0.22%-Caryophyllene oxide, 0.20%-Limonene, 0.19%-Bornyl formate,0.18%-beta-Pinene, 0.16%-delta-3-Carene,0.15%-trans-Pinocarveol, 0.11%-para-Cymene,0.09%-Eugenol, 0.09%-Isoborneol, 0.07%-Myrcene,0.07%-Spathulenol, 0.06%-beta-Bisabolene, 0.06%-alpha-Bergamotene, 0.05%-alpha-Copaene, 0.05%-cis-Jasmone, 0-04%-alpha-Humulene,0.04%-beta-Bourbonene, 0.03%-Tricyclene,0.03%-(E)-beta-Ocimene, 0.03%-Camphor, 0.03%-Myrtenal, 0.02%-Sabinene, 0.02%-alpha-Terpineol, 0.02%-cis-Sabinene hydrate, 0.02%-(Z)-3-Hexenol, 0.02%-(Z)-3-Hexenyl acetate, 0.01%-Terpinolene, 0.01%-alpha-Muurolene, 0.01%-Fenchone, 0.01%-alpha-Farnesene, 0.01%-alpha-Fenchene, 0.01%-2-Hexenal, 0.01%-Acetone, 0.01%-2-Butanone, 0.01%-Octane
- 1.2% to 25.1%-beta-Caryophyllene, 63.0% to 92.9%-Precocene I
- Precocene I, beta-Caryophyllene
- 43.99%-Precocene II, 23.34%-Precocene I, 9.18%-beta-Caryophyllene,2.67%-beta-Cubebene,2.15%-beta-Gurjunene,

1.97%-Geranial, 1.63%-Geraniol, 1.32%-Camphene, 1.31%-Neral, 1.18%-Bornylacetate, 0.98%-(E)-beta-Farnesene, 0.95%-Sesquiterpenes, oxygen-containing-, 0.68%-alpha-Phellandrene, 0.65%-Sesquiterpenehydrocarbon(unknown), 0.61%-Epibicyclosesquiphellandrene, 0.51%-Geranyl acetat, 0.49%-alpha-Humulene, 0.33%-Demethoxyencecalin, 0.30%-Androencecalinol, 0.26%-(Z)-beta-Ocimene, 0.24%-Caryophyllene oxide, 0.22%-Myrcene, 0.21%-Nerol, 0.21%-alpha-Cubebene, 0.21%-(E)-Nerolidol, 0,20%-alpha-Farnesene, 0.19%-alpha-Pinene, 0.19%-para-Cymene, 0.18%-alpha-Copaene 0.17%-2-Carene, 0.16%-(E)-beta-Ocimene, 0.15%-beta-Pinene, 0.14%-Eupatoriochromene, 0.13%-Neryl acetate, 0.13%-alpha-Muurolene, 0.11%-Linalool, 0.10% Undecane, 0.08%-Borneol, 0.01%-gamma-Terpinene, 0.01%-alpha-Ylangene, 0.01%-alpha-Gurjunen, 0.01%-(Z)-beta-Farnesene, 0.01%-Hexadecanoic acid, 0.01%-Bornyl formate, 0.01%-Tetradecanoic acid, 0.01%-beta-Bourbonene, 0.01%-Germacrene B, 0.01%-Oleic acid 0.01%-Octadecanoic acid, 0.01%-2-Methylnaphthalene, 0.01%-Dimethylnaphthalene (unknown isomer)

2. *Ageratum haustonianum* Miller.- Herb to 1 m, annual, hairy. Leaves serrate, acuminate, corymb dense, capitula blue. Flowers deep blue. (often higher altitude specimens of A.conyzoides, with progressively larger and deeper blue capitula, are confused with this species).

Major Essential Oil

- alpha-Farnesene – 46.6%, alpha-Farnesene, Germacrene-D – 18.16%, delta-Cadinene – 3.7%
- 43.99%-Precocene II, 23.34%-Precocene I, 9.18%-beta-Caryophyllene, 2.67%-beta-Cubebene, 2.15%-beta-Gurjunene, 1.97%-Geranial, 1.63%-Geraniol, 1.32%-Camphene, 1.31%-Neral, 1.18%-Bornylacetate, 0.98%-(E)-beta-Farnesene, 0.95%-Sesquiterpenes, oxygen-containing-, 0.68%-alpha-Phellandrene, 0.65%-Sesquiterpene hydrocarbons (unknown), 0.61%-Epibicyclosesquiphellandrene, 0.51%-Geranyl acetat, 0.49%-alpha-Humulene, 0.33%-

Demethoxyencecalin, 0.30%-Androencecalinol, 0.26%-(Z)-beta-Ocimene, 0.24%-Caryophyllene oxide, 0.22%-Myrcene, 0.21%-Nerol, 0.21%-alpha-Cubebene, 0.21%-(E)-Nerolidol, 0,20%-alpha-Farnesene, 0.19%-alpha-Pinene, 0.19%-para-Cymene, 0.18%-alpha-Copaene, 0.17%-2-Carene, 0.16%-(E)-beta-Ocimene, 0.15%-beta-Pinene, 0.14%-Eupatoriochromene, 0.13%-Nerylacetate, 0.13%-alpha-Muurolene, 0.11%-Linalool, 0.10%-Undecane, 0.08%-Borneol, 0.01%-gamma-Terpinene, 0.01%-alpha-Ylangene, 0.01%-alpha-Gurjunen, 0.01%-(Z)-beta-Farnesene, 0.01%-Hexadecanoic acid, 0.01%-Bornyl formate, 0.01%-Tetradecanoic acid, 0.01%-beta-Bourbonene, 0.01%-Germacrene B, 0.01%-Oleic acid0.01%-Octadecanoic acid, 0.01%-2-Methylnaphthalene, 0.01%-Dimethylnaphthalene (unknownisomer)

3. *Chromolaena odorata* (Linn) R.King & H. Robinson. (*Eupatorium odoratum*. Linn.)- Aromatic, erect, viscid – pubescent sub shrub to 3 m. Leaves opposite, simple obovate, to deltoid ovate, acute, crenate, serrate, sub palmately 3 nerved. Capitula corymbose, stalked corolla white to purple. Flowers homogamous.

Value Added Property

- As antiseptic and to heal wounds — Plant
- Antibacterial — Essential oil

Major Essential Oil

- beta-Caryophyllene – 21.5%, Carvacrol – 11.01%, alpha-Pinene-5.4%, Thymol – 3.3%, beta-Pinene – 2.7%, Limonene – 0.5%
- 18.8%-alpha-Pinene, 14.3%-Pregeijerene10.5%-beta Pinene

4. *Eupotorium triplinerve* Vahl. (*E.ayapana* Vent.)- An aromatic under shrub, 0.9 – 1.2 m high with trailing stem, rooting at the nodes. Subsessile lanceolate leaves and lax corymbs of bluish flower heads. Flowers homogamous.

Value Added Property

Use	Part
• As tonic	Plant
• In ulcers, sores and to bite of venomous reptiles	Plant and leaves
• In various kinds of haemorrhages	Leaves
• As cardiac stimulant increasing the force of the heart beat	Leaves
• As expectorant, diaphorectic and antiperiodic	Leaves and flowering tops and twig
• In cholera and yellow fever	Infusion
• Bitter, astringent, acrid thermogenic, stimulant, digestive, carminative, alterant, emetic and purgative in large doses. Haemostatic, vulnerary, cardiotonic, antiscorbutic, alexeteric, sudorific, antipyretic, detergent, anti inflammatory, expetorant and tonic and is useful in gastropathy, dyspepsia, epistaxis, haematomesis, haemorrhages, haemoptysis, haematuria, menorrhagia, haemorrhoides, wounds ulcers, ulcerative stomatitis, cardiac debility. Skin eruptions, scabies, pruitus, poison bites, intermittent fevers especially yellow fever, inflammation, cough, asthma, vitiated conditions of kapha and general debility.	Plant

Major Essential Oil

- Thymohydroquinone dimethyl ether, coumarin

5. *Mikania cordata* (Burm.F) Robins. (*M. scandens*, Willd.)—The plant is a climbing shrub, leaves long petioled, ovate, acute or acuminate base rounded cordate or truncate crenate or angled. Some times villous beneath. Heads 4 flowered corymbose terminating lateral branches, homogamous.

Major Essential Oil

- beta-Caryophyllene – 18.5%, Thymol – 12.4%, alpha-Pinene – 3.5%, beta-Pinene – 0.9%, Germacrene-D – 0.63%.

6. *Conyza bonariensis* (Linn) Cronq.- Sericeous herb. Leaves linear – lanceolate, hirsute above and below, margin entire

to sparingly serrate, sub sessile, panicles terminal lax racemose, capitula cream.

Major Essential Oil

- alpha-Humulene – 35.2%, beta-Caryophyllene – 6.13%, alpha-Farnesene- 2.8%, Limonene – 0.96%

7. *Conyza canadensis* (Linn) Cronq.-It is an annual plant with an erect branched stem, densely covered with narrowly lance-shaped leaves, and bearing many flower heads in dense clusters. Each flower heads has many central tubular disk florets and several outer rows of ray florets. Both are yellow and white.

Major Essential Oil

- alpha-Humulene – 25.3%, beta-Caryophyllene – 8.3%, delta-Cadinene – 2.9%.

8. *Blumea lacera* DC.- Strongly scented herb to 75 cm, glandular pubescent, interspersed with eglandular hairs. Leaves elliptic oblanceolate, 2.5 – 6 x 1.3 – 3.5 cm capitula 5 – 7, shortly stalked in dense corymbose, spiciform, panicles terminating the branchlets. Corolla yellow in disc florets.

Value Added Property

- As insect repellent, anti bacterial and anti fungal Essential oil
- As vegetable — Leaves
- Astringent, diuretic and febrifugal anthelmintic particularly in the case of thread worm; in bleeding piles — Juice
- In cholera to relieve dryness in the mouth — Roots

Major Essential Oil

- alpha-Humulene – 11.08%, beta-Selinene – 10.4%, beta-Caryophyllene – 5.2%, Germacrene-D – 4.3%, delta-Cadinene – 4.2%, Eugenol – 1.4%, Terpinen-4-ol – 0.4%
- 66%-Cineol, 10%-defenchone , 6%-Citral
- alpha-Pinene, beta-Pinene, beta-Bisabolene

9. *Blumea mollis* (D.Don) Merr.- Villous silky hairy, stems erect sub simple very leafy, leaves petioled, obovate, irregularly toothed. Head 0.6 cm collected into terminal spiciform dense cymes. Heads heterogamous. Corolla purple.

Value Added Property

- Anti bacterial and Anti fungal Essential oil

Major Essential Oil

- Linalyl acetate – 26.3%, beta-Caryophyllene – 18.2%, beta-Bisabolene – 17.3%, delta-Cadinene – 2.8%
- Cadinene, Camphene, Cymene,Caryophyllene, Humulene, beta-Terpinene, 1,8 Cineol, Linalool, Linalyl acetate, Isoborneol, Caryophyllene oxide

10. *Sphaeranthus indicus* Linn.- The plant is an annual herb with spreading branch, leaves alternate, toothed, decurrent on the stem. Heads small heterogamous not rayed. Pink or purple flowers, collected together in close terminal globose clusters.

Value Added Property

Property	Part
• Bitter, stomachic, stimulant, alterative, pectoral and dimolcent and externally emollient	Plant
• Stomachic and anthelmintic	Roots and Seeds
• In worms and indigestion	Plant
• Styptic, in liver and gastric disorders and in itch	Juice
• In chest pains, cough and bowel complaints	Root
• In piles	Barks
• Alterative, depurative and tonic property	Flower
• In cough	Leaves
• Anti tubercular property	Plant
• The leaves are eaten as pot herb. They are mixed with paddy and rice to prevent damage by insect, pests, during storage. The herb is employed as a fish poison. It is also stuffed into holes of crabs to kill them.	Plant

Major Essential Oil

- alpha-Humulene – 14.1%, delta-Cadinene – 12.5%, beta-Caryophyllene – 10.8%, beta-Selinene – 9.85%, beta-Ionone – 5.5%
- 12.6%-alpha-Ionone, 7.4%-beta-Caryophyllene, 7.4%-para-Methoxycinnamaldehyde, 7.0%-Eugenol, 2.2%-alpha-Terpinene, 15.3%-Cadinene, 6.7%-Ocimene
- 15.3%-Cadinene, 12.6%-alpha-Ionone, 7.4%-beta-Caryophyllene, 7.4%-p-methoxycinnamaldehyde, 7.0%-Eugenol,7.0%-alpha-Phellandrene, 6.1%-Ocimene, 5.4%-Citral, 2.2%-alpha-Terpinene, and an unidentified sesquiterpene (b.p127 – 28/10mm)
- Methyl chavicol, alpha-Ionone, delta-Candinene, para-Methoxycinnamaldehyde, Ocimene, alpha-Terpinene, Citral, Geraniol, Geranyl acetate, beta-Ionone

11. *Bidens pilosa* Linn.- The plant is a very variable erect herb, leaves 3 fid – 3 foliate. Heads on long stout peduncles very variable in length, with white rays. Heads heterogamous.

Major Essential Oil

- beta-Caryophyllene – 27.44%, beta-Bisabolene – 20.0%, alpha-Humulene – 6.46%, beta-Elemene – 3.08%, Germacrene-D – 1.05%
- 25.00%-Germacrene D, 20.00%-1-Phenylhepta-1,3,5-triyne,18.00%-beta-Caryophyllene, 8.00%-alpha-Pinene, 5.60%-Bicyclogermacrene, 3.50%-beta-Copaene, 3.00%-delta-Cadinene, 1.90%-alpha-Humulene,1.60%-Limonene, 1.20%-T-Muurolol, 1.00%-beta-Pinene,1.00%-beta-Elemene, 1.00%-Nerolidol (unknown isomer),1.00%-alpha-Cadinol,1.00%-(E)-beta-Farnesene,0.90%-Linalool, 0.80%-gamma-Cadinene, 0.80%-Farnesene(unknown isomer), 0.70%-alpha-Muurolene, 0.70%-alpha-Copaene, 0.50%-Precocene 1, 0.40%-Myrcene, 0.30%, Caryophyllene oxide, 0.25%-alpha-Terpineol, 0.20%-Spathulenol, 0.10%-(Z)-beta-Ocimene, 0.10%-alpha-Ylangene, 0.05%-Camphene,0.05%-Sabinene, 0.05%-alpha-

Phellandrene, 0.05%-(E)-beta-Ocimene, 0.05%-gamma-Terpinene, 0.05%-Terpinolene, 0.05%-Terpinen-4-01, 0.05%-1,8-Cineole

12. *Cosmos bipinnatus* Cav. cv. Orange.- Tall herbs, to 80 cm high, leaves 2 – 4 pinnatisect, lobes entire, glabrous, 7 – 8 cm long. Peduncle long ligules orange red to yellow, sometimes white; disc florets orange in colour. Grown in gardens, occurring as escape and naturalizing in plains and upper ghats.

Major Essential Oil

- alpha-Humulene – 26.8%, delta-Cadinene – 5.78%, Germacrene-D – 4.39%, beta-Caryophyllene – 2.35%, Terpenen-4-ol – 0.37%

13. *Cosmos bipinnatus* Cav. cv. Yellow.- Erect herbs, leaves long, opposite, bipinnatisect, petioles upto 2.5 cm long sheating at base, Heads terminal, Disc florets yellow.

Major Essential Oil

- alpha-Humulene – 23.4%,delta-Cadinene – 4.89%, Germacrene-D – 2.23%, beta-Caryophyllene – 1.95%

14. *Cosmos caudatus* Kunth.- Erect annual herb 0.5 – 1.5 m tall. Leaves bipinnatisect or some what tripinnatisect, pinnules opposite, capitulam solitary, axillary or terminal, long stalked, heterogamous,corolla purple.

Major Essential Oil

- alpha-Humulene – 26.8%, Germacrene-D – 11.25%, delta-Cadinene – 9.8%, beta-Caryophyllene – 1.8%, Linalyl acetate – 0.39%, Limonene – 0.16%

15. *Parthenium hysterophorus* Linn-The plant is a herb. 1.0 m in height, stem long; tridinally grooved, leaves irregularly dissected, head is corymbose head; homogamous white flowers.

Major Essential Oil

- delta-Cadinene – 19.78%, beta-Caryophyllene – 5.98%, alpha-Pinene – 4.09%

Value Added Property

- As tonic, febrifuge, emmenagogue and analgesic in neuralgia — Plant
- In dysentery — Roots

16. *Spilanthes ciliata* H.B.K (*S. acmella* Murr.)-Diffuse herbs rooting at lower nodes. Stem terete. Leaves to 7 x 4 cm ovate, base rounded or sub cordate margins serrate, apex acute, petiole 1 – 2.5 cm long. Heads rayed axillary, usually solitary, rarely 2 –3 in each axil, turning conical, yellow, peduncle 3 –8 cm long. Involucral bracts 2 seriate shorter than ray florets.

Value Added Property

- In toothache and affections of throat and gums and paralysis of the tongue, dysentery, rheumatism — Flower head
- In dysentery — Plant
- As diuertic and lithontriptic and is employed both for rheumatism and as a lotion in scabies and psoriasis — Decoction
- In wounds — Herb powder

Major Essential Oil

- beta-Caryophyllene – 19.36%, delta-Cadinene – 10.97%, Germacrene-D – 8.0%, alpha-Humulene – 6.6%, beta-Selinene – 5.6%, Methyl chavicol – 5.3%, Thymol – 5.0%.
- 23.6%-Limonene, 20.9%-beta-Caryophyllene, 10.8%-Germacrene D.
- 30.24%-beta-Caryophyllene, 18.30%-Thymol, 13.34%-gamma-Cadinene, 8.43%-(Z)-beta-Ocimene, 4.68%-beta-Phellandrene, 3.06%-gamma-Elemene, 2.90%-beta-Pinene, 2.59%-Sesquiterpene hydrocarbons (unknown), 2.46%-alpha-Humulene, 2.20%-Myrcene, 1.96%-delta-Cadinene, 1.47%-para-Cymene, 1.42%-alpha-Copaene, 1.11%-Sabinene, 1.10%-

Methyl chavicol, 0.41%-beta-Selinene 0.39%-alpha-Pinene, 0.23%-(E)-beta-Ocimene

17. *Synedrella nodiflora*, Gaertn.- The plant is an erect dichotomously branched herb, stem and branches terette, glabrous, leaves ovate lanceolate, shortly petioled serrate, scaberulous, 3 nerved. Heads sessile, axillary and terminal. Heads small heterogamous, flowers yellow.

Value Added Property

- As prultice for sore legs and for the preparation of embrocation for rheumatism — Leaves

Major Essential Oil

- Farnesene – 22.75%, beta-Caryophyllene – 12.7%, delta-Cadinene – 2.35%,

  Germacrene-D – 1.27%, Limonene – 0.27%, beta-Pinene – 0.2%, alpha- Pinene – 0.03%

- 43.96%-beta-Caryophyllene, 11.93%-beta-Farnesene, 7.64%-Germacrene D, 6.68%-beta-Cubebene, 2.93%-Sesquiterpene hydrocarbons (unknown), 2.48%-Caryophyllene oxide, 2.15%-(Z)-3-Hexenol, 2.01%-1-Hexanol, 1.91%-Myrcene, 1.91%-Sesquiterpene alcohols (unknown), 1.43%-alpha-Copaene, 1.37%-beta-Bourbonene, 1.37%-Bicyclogermacrene, 1.05%-(E)-2-Hexenol, 1.03%-Limonene, 0.95%-delta-Cadinene, 0.71%-delta-Elemene, 0.69%-beta-Elemene, 0.50%-alpha-Cubebene, 0.29%-gamma-Elemene, 0.21%-beta-Pinene, 0.12%-alpha-Pinene, 0.12%-Calamenene, 0.01%-Camphene, 0.01%-para-Cymene, 0.01%-Monoterpene hydrocarbons

18. *Wedelia chinensis* (Osbeck) Merrill (*W. Calendulacea* Less.)- It is a climbing shrub. Leaves linear-oblong or oblanceolate, sub sessile, entire, roughly scabrous, heads solitary on slender axillary peduncles 5 – 12.5 cm long. Head heterogamous with yellow ray flowers.

Value Added Property

- Astringent, bitter, acrid, thermogenic, anti-inflammatory, vulnerary ophthalmic, cardic tonic, anthelmintic, diuretic, aphrodisiae, sudorific, febrifuge and trichogenous.

- In vitiated conditions of kapha and vata, inflammation, elephantiasis otalgia, cephalalgia, wounds, ulcers, nyctalopia, dysopia, hepato plenomegaly, colic, dyspepsia, helminthiasis, strangury, anaemia, seminal weakness, fever, baldness and greyness of hair and is very specific for viral hepatitis — Plant
- As tonic and alterative useful in cough, cephalagia and diseases, of skin, especially alopecia. — Plant
- In uterine haemorrhage and urenorrhagia — Plant
- For dyeing grey hair, and for promoting their growth their
- Their juice is used for tattoing — Plant
- In cuts, ulcers, sores and varicose veins — Leaf powder
- In stomach ache — Root

19. *Wedelia trilobata* (Linn) Hitch—It is a climbing shrub scabrid pubescent or hirsute herbs or under shrubs, leaves opposite, trilobed often triple nerved. Heads heterogamous rayed, axillary or terminal, radiate, yellow flowers.

Major Essential Oil

- alpha-Pinene – 23.7%, beta-Pinene – 21.99%,Thymol – 12.7%, beta-Caryophyllene – 5.26%, Limonene – 5.21%, beta-Phellandrene – 3.65%
- 30.30%-alpha-Pinene, 17.40%-alpha-Phellandrene,16.30%-Limonene, 6.40%-beta-Pinene, 5.30%-gamma-Muurolene, 2.80%-Camphene,2.60%-Myrcene, 2.60%-(E)-beta-Ocimene, 2.46%-gamma-Elemene, 2.30%-(Z)-beta-Ocimene, 2.30%-beta-Caryophyllene, 1.80%-alpha-Humulene, 0.01%-Thymol, 0.01%-Carvacrol

20. *Tagetes erecta* Linn cv. orange-A stout branching herb, 60 cm tall, leaves strong scented, pinnately dissected segments 1 – 5 cm long oblong or lanceolate, serrate, flower heads solitary, orange in colour, rays many long clawed.

Value Added Property

- Purgative — Roots and seeds
- Antiseptic, and a fly repellent — Oil
- In cuts and wounds — Juice
- As carminative — Flowers
- Fungitoxic propery against pathogenic fungi — Plant

Major Essential Oil

- Linalool – 34.5%, Limonene – 21.95%, beta-Caryophyllene – 20.36%, Piperitone – 3.13%, beta-Pinene – 2.96%, Sabinene – 1.29%, alpha-Pinene – 0.36%
- 30.30%-alpha-Pinene, 17.40%-alpha-Phellandrene, 16.30%-Limonene, 6.40%-beta-Pinene, 5.30%-gamma-Muurolene, 2.80%-Camphene, 2.60%-Myrcene, 2.60%-(E)-beta-Ocimene, 2.46%-gamma-Elemene, 2.30%-(Z)-beta-Ocimene, 2.30%-beta-Caryophyllene, 1.80%-alpha-Humulene, 0.01%-Thymol, 0.01%-Carvacrol
- 20.02%-Piperitone, 13.13%-(E)-beta-Ocimene,12.41%-Terpinolene, 11.02%-Limonene, 4.44%-Thymol, 3.60%-beta-Caryophyllene, 3.16%-(Z)-beta-Ocimene, 2.85%-Indole, 2.70%-Piperitenone, 2.08%-Nerolidol (unknown isomer), 2.01%-Myrcene, 1.65%-(E)-beta-Farnesene,1.51%-Sabinene, 1.02%-Carvacrol,1.02%-1,3,8-p-Menthatriene, 0.78%-alpha-Pinene, 0.65%-Linalool, 0.39%-p-Cymen-8-ol, 0-39%-gamma-Elemene, 0.36%-Geranyl acetate, 0.33%-Cyperene, 0.28%-Terpinen-4-ol, 0.26%-gamma-Terpinene, 0.18%-beta-Elemene,0.16%-gamma-Muurolene, 0.09%-Camphene, 0.07%-beta-Pinene
- 18.30%-Limonene, 15.30%-(E)-beta-Ocimene, 15.30%-beta-Caryophyllene, 15.30%-Piperitone

21. *Tagetes patula* Linn.-Sub shrub to 1m. Stem dark red in colour, leaves aromatic, alternate, pinnate, capitulam solitary, terminal or axillary, heterogamous, corolla orange red in colour Thymol – 23.65%

Major Essential Oil

- Sabinene – 11.29%, beta-Caryophyllene – 6.19%, beta-Phellandrene – 5.96%, Limonene – 4.18%, Linalool – 3.38%, beta-Pinene – 0.97%, Piperitone – 0.64%, alpha-Pinene – 0.37%
- 14.20% -Limonene,13.40% -(Z)-Ocimenone,13.40%-(E)-Ocimenone,11.90%-beta Caryophyllene,11.70%-(E) –beta Ocimene,7.00%-(E)-Tageto,3.40%- Nerol.

22. *Emilia sonchifolia* (Linn) Dc.- The plant is a small herb, stems and leaves soft, fistular, glauceous, glabrous or nearly so, the leaves lyrate pinnatifed with large terminal lobe, upto 10 cm long the basal leaves petioled cauline, accurately auricled corolla lobes very short. Head small. Homogenous.

Value Added Property

• Astringent, sweet, thermogenic, sudorific, antipyretic, ophthalmic, vulnerary, anti-asthmatic and is used in vitiated conditions of vata, infantile tympanities, gastropathy, diarrhoea, otalgia, ophthlmia, nyctalopia, cuts and wounds, intermittent fevers, pharyngodynia and asthma	Plant
• As febrifuge in infantile tympanites and in bowel complaints	Plant
• In diarrhoea	Roots
• In sore ears, sore eyes and night blindness	Leaves
• In cuts and wounds	Plant

Major Essential Oil

- alpha-Humulene – 28.5%, beta-Caryophyllene – 11.98%, beta-Bisabolene – 6.45%, Germacrene-D – 4.15%, Terpenen-4-ol – 1.56%, Linalool – 0.15%

23. *Notonia grandiflora* Dc.- Plant is a fleshy shrub reaching 1.5 m in height, with pale yellow flowers, turning green. Leaves obovate or oblanceolate or sub orbicular, obtuse, variable in size but some times reaching 17 cm long and 8 cm broad, quite entire glacious green heads 2.0 cm – 3.0 cm long. Head large, homogamous not rayed all bisexual in long peduncled corymbs.

Value Added Property

- As cure for pimples Plant

Major Essential Oil

- alpha-Humulene – 13%, beta-Caryophyllene – 12.2%, delta-Cadinene 11.5%, alpha-Pinene – 0.1%

3

Chemical Composition of the Essential Oil of Asteraceae

Achillea Abrotanoides

BOTANICAL SPECIES

Achillea abrotanoides (Vis.) Vis., fam. Asteraceae (Compositae)

AUTHOR

Bicchi, C., Frattini, C., and Cantamessa, L.

TITLE

On the Composition of Achillea abrotanoides (Vis.). Vis. Essential Oil

PUBLICATION

Flavour Fragr. J., Vol. 3, (3), 101-104 (1988)

COMPOUNDS

18.50%	-	1,8-Cineole
14.20%	-	Camphor
10.90%	-	Camphene
10.20%	-	beta-Thujone

9.40%	-	Bornyl acetate	
7.60%	-	para-Cymene	
5.50%	-	alpha-Thujene	
5.50%	-	Terpinen-4-ol	
4.10%	-	gamma-Terpinene	
2.90%	-	Sabinene	
1.10%	-	beta-Pinene	
0.90%	-	alpha-Pinene	
0.50%	-	Borneol	
0.40%	-	alpha-Terpmene	
0.30%	-	alpha-Thujone	
0.20%	-	alpha-Terpineol	
0.05%	-	cis-Piperitol	
0.05%	-	trans-Piperitol	
0.05%	-	Þ-Cymen-8-ol	
0.05%	-	Thymol	
92.50		TOTAL %	20 COMPOUNDS

Achillea biebersteinii (Turkey) 1

BOTANICAL SPECIES

Achillea biebersteinii Afan., fam. Asteraceae (Compositae)

AUTHOR

Chialva,F.,Monguzzi, F., Manitto,P. and Akgul,A.

TITLE

Essntial Oil Constituets of Achillea biebersteinii Afan.
(0.01%=trace)

PUBLICATION

J. Essent.Oil Res.,Vol. 5,87-88(Jan/Feb 1993)

COMPOUNDS

46.18%	-	1, 8-Cineole
17.61%	-	Camphor
8.23%	-	alpha-Terpineol
3.41%	-	Borneol
3.18%	-	Sabinene
3.06%	-	Terpinen-4-ol
1.88%	-	alpha-Pinene
1.49%	-	Camphene
1.41%	-	Ocimenol
1.35%	-	beta-Pinene
0.94%	-	trans-Sabinene hydrate
0.73%	-	cis-Sabinene hydrate
0.73%	-	ganma-Muurolene
0.54%	-	beta-Eudesmol
0.44%	-	Bornyl acetate
0.42%	-	Myrtenol
0.40%	-	Methyl chavicol
0.30%	-	Linalool
0.26%	-	Eugenol

0.25%	-	Pinocarvone
0.24%	-	trans-Pinocarveol
0.24%	-	Caryophyllene oxide
0.22%	-	para-Cymene
0.22%	-	Myrtenal
0.22%	-	dehydro-1, 8-Cineole
0.19%	-	Geraniol
0.18%	-	Carvone
0.17%	-	cis-Piperitol
0.15%	-	Cumin alcohol
0.14%	-	(E)-Anethole
0.13%	-	Limonene
0.12%	-	Thymol
0.11%	-	trans-Piperitol
0.11%	-	Methyl eugenol
0.01%	-	Tricyclene
0.01%	-	alpha-Thujene
0.01%	-	Myrcene
0.01%	-	alpha-Terpinene
0.01%	-	gamma-Terpinene
0.01%	-	Terpinolene
0.01%	-	beta-Caryophyllene
0.01%	-	Carvacrol
0.01%	-	(E)-Nerolidol
0.01%	-	cis-Carveol
0.01%	-	p-Methoxyphenylacetone
0.01%	-	Cuminaldehyde
0.01%	-	cis-Jasmone
95.38	TOTAL %	47 COMPOUNDS

Achillea biebersteinii (Turkey) 2

BOTANICAL SPECIES

Achillea biebersteinii Afan., fam. Asteraceae (Compositae)

AUTHOR

Kuesmenoglu S., et al.

TITLE

Constituents of the Essential Oil of Achillea biebersteinii Afan. (average of 2 samples from different areas in Turkey)

PUBLICATION

J. Essent. Oil Res, Vol. 7, 527-528 (Sep/Oct 1995)

COMPOUNDS

26.65%	-	Piperitone
20.40%	-	1,8-Cineole
13.25%	-	Camphor
3.50%	-	alpha-Terpinyl acetate
2.05%	-	para-Cymene
2.00%	-	alpha-Terpineol
1.55%	-	Camphene
1.24%	-	alpha-Pinene
1.15%	-	Terpinen-4-ol
0.90%	-	Chrysanthenone
0.70%	-	Borneol
0.68%	-	p-Cymen-8-ol
0.56%	-	Germacrene D
0.55%	-	beta-Pinene
0.55%	-	Myrtenol
0.50%	-	cis-Piperitol
0.50%	-	Carveol

0.46%	-	trans-Pinocarveol
0.45%	-	alpha-Terpinene
0.44%	-	Cuminaldehyde
0.40%	-	Jasmone
0.40%	-	cis-Carveol
0.32%		cis-Sabinene hydrate
0.31%	-	Bornyl acetate
0.29%		cis-p-Mentha-2,8-dien-1-ol
0.28%	-	gamma-Terpinene
0.25%	-	(E,Z)-2,4-Decadienal
0.24%	-	Limonene
0.21%	-	Sabinene
0.21%	-	Carvone
0.19%	-	Grandisol
0.14%	-	Cumin alcohol
0.14%	-	Santolina alcohol
0 13%	-	Carvacrol
0.12%	-	Campholene aldehyde
0.11%	-	trans-Verbenol
0.10%	-	Eugenol
0.10%	-	Caryophyllene oxide
0.10%	-	Chrysanthenyl acetate
0.10%	-	p-Mentha-1,3-dien-7-ol
0.08%	-	Tricyclene
0.07%	-	(E)-2-Hexenal
0.06%	-	Hexanal
0.05%	-	alpha-Phellandrene
0.05%	-	Terpinolene
0.05%	-	Thymol
0,05%	-	6,10,14-Trimethyl-2-pentadecanone
0.03%	-	Nonanal

0.03%	-	Spathulenol
0.03%	-	(E)-2-Hexenol
0.02%	-	Myrcene
0.02%	-	1-Hexanol
0.01%	-	alpha-Thujone
0.01%	-	2-Pentylfuran
0.01%	-	(Z)-3-Hexenol
0.01%	-	2-Ethylfuran
0.01%	-	3-Methylpentanal
0.01%	-	3,5,5-Trimethyl-2 -cyclohexen-1-ol
82.82		TOTAL % 58 COMPOUNDS

Achillea collina

BOTANICAL SPECIES

Achillea collina Becker, fam. Asteraceae (Compositae)

AUTHOR

Mishurova S.S. et al.

TITLE

Chemical Composition of Achillea collina oil

PUBLICATION

Rastit. Resur. 21, 69-73 (1985); [(C.A. Vol. 102, 128858c (1985)]

COMPOUNDS

33.80%	-	beta-Pinene
19.20%	-	Bornyl acetate
13.20%	-	Chamazulenes (unknown structure)
8.10%	-	beta-Caryophyllene
7.70%	-	1,8-Cineole
6.80%	-	Borneol
3.20%	-	alpha-Pinene
2.90%	-	Cadinene (unknown isomer)
2.20%	-	Camphor
2.20%	-	ortho-Cymene
0.40%	-	Camphene
0.05%	-	para-Cymene
0.05%	-	Linalool
99.80	TOTAL %	13 COMPOUNDS

Achillea ligustica flower (Greece)

BOTANICAL SPECIES

Achillea ligustica All., fam. Asteraceae (Compositae)

AUTHOR

Tzakou, O., Loukis, A., Verykokidou, E., and Roussis, V.

TITLE

Chemical Constituents of the Essential Oil of Achillea ligustica All. from Greece

PUBLICATION

J. Essent. Oil Res., Vol. 7, 549-550 (Sep/Oct 1995)

COMPOUNDS

70.84%	-	Linalool
6.98%	-	1, 8-Cineoie
2.01%	-	Piperitone
1.48%	-	alpha-Terpineol
1.06%	-	Terpinen-4-ol
0.96%	-	beta-Pinene
0.90%	-	cis-p-Menth-2-en-1-ol
0.88%	-	Limonene
0.68%	-	Borneol
0.46%	-	Pinocarvone
0.44%	-	trans-Linalool oxide (5) (furanoid)
0.38%	-	Sabinene
0 33%	-	alpha-Pinene
0.29%	-	gamma-Terpinene
0.29%	-	Nerolidol (unknown isomer)
0.28%	-	Alloocimene (unknown isomer)
0.26%	-	beta-Caryophyllene

0.25%	-	Viridiflorol
0.22%	-	Myrcene
0.21%	-	cis-Jasmone
0.20%	-	Camphor
0.19%	-	Germacrene D
0.18%	-	delta-3-Carene
0.16%	-	Geraniol
0.16%	-	gamma-Terpineol
0.13%	-	1,3,8-p-Menthatriene
0.11%	-	para-Cymeme
0.11%	-	Myrtenol
0.10%	-	delta-Cadinene
0.09%	-	Camphene
0.09%	-	alpha-Phellandrene
0.06%	-	Nerol
0.06%	-	Bornyl acetate
0.06%	-	Verbenone
0.05%	-	Aromadendrene
0.04%	-	Terpinolene
0.04%	-	alpha-Cubebene
0.03%	-	alpha-Thujene
0.03%	-	Neryl acetate
0.02%	-	Isoborneol
0.01%	-	alpha-Thujone
0.01%	-	Myrtenal
91.13	TOTAL %	42 COMPOUNDS

Achillea ligustica leaf (Greece)

BOTANICAL SPECIES

Achillea ligustica All., fam. Asteraceae (Compositae)

AUTHOR

Tzakou, O., Loukis, A., Verykokidou, E., and Roussis, A.

TITLE

Chemical Constituents of the Essential Oil of Achillea ligustica All. from Greece

PUBLICATION

J. Essent. Oil Res., Vol. 7, 549-550 (Sep/Oct 1995)

COMPOUNDS

28.15%	-	Linalool
4.57%	-	1, 8-Cineole
2.83%	-	Piperitone
1.42%	-	Viridiflorol
1.36%	-	beta-Pinene
1.13%	-	alpha-Terpineol
1.04%	-	Pinocarvone
0.80%	-	Terpinen-4-ol
0.76%	-	(E)-Nerolidol
0.60%	-	beta-Caryophyllene
0.55%	-	1, 3, 8-p-Menthatriene
0.54%	-	Sabinene
0, 53%	-	Camphor
0.47%	-	Borneol
0.46%	-	delta-Cadinene
0.46%	-	Alloocimene (unknown isomer)
0.45%	-	trans-Linalool oxide (5) (furanoid)

0.43%	-	Myrtenol
0.42%	-	cis-Jasmone
0.35%	-	alpha-Pinene
0.35%	-	gamma-Terpineol
0.32%	-	cis-p-Menth-2-en-1-ol
0.25%	-	para-Cymene
0.22%	-	gamma-Terpinene
0.20%	-	Myrtenal
0.18%	-	Myrcene
0.17%	-	delta-3-Carene
0.16%	-	Limonene
0.16%	-	beta-Cubebene
0.16%		trans-Pinocarvyl acetate
0.13%	-	alpha-Copaene
0.10%	-	Neryl acetate
0.09%	-	alpha-Thujone
0.09%	-	Aromadendrene
0.07%	-	alpha-Phellandrene
0.07%	-	Terpinolene
0.07%	-	Bornyl acetate
0.07%	-	Isoborneol
0.04%	-	alpha-Thujene
0.04%	-	Camphene
50.26		TOTAL % 40 COMPOUNDS

Achillea wilhelmsii (Egypt)

BOTANICAL SPECIES

Achillea wilhelmsii C. Koch (A. santolina Auct. Mult.), fam. Asteraceae

AUTHOR

Brunke, E.-J., Hammerschmidt, F.-J., and AboutabI, E.A.

TITLE

Volatile Constituents of Achiilea Wilhelmsii C. Koch (syn. A. Santolina Auct. Mult.) from Egypt and the Turkey

PUBLICATION

In: Progress in Essential Oil Research (Proc. Intern. Symp. on Ess. Oils), E.-J. Brunke, Ed., Walter de Gruyter, Berlin (1986), 85-97

COMPOUNDS

25.50%	-	trans-Fragranyl acetate
15.00%	-	Camphor
13.70%	-	1,8-Cineole
9.10%	-	Fragranol
6.90%	-	Terpinen-4-ol
3.90%	-	para-Cymene
1.90%	-	Camphene
1.50%	-	alpha-Thujone
1.10%	-	cis-Sabinene hydrate
1.00%	-	trans-Sabinene hydrate
1.00%	-	Caryophylladienols
0.90%	-	alpha-Pinene
0.60%	-	Sabinene
0.60%	-	alpha-Terpineol
0.50%	-	gamma-Terpinene

0.50%	-	Borneol
0.50%	-	Fragranyl 2-methylbutyrate
0.50%	-	dehydro-1, 8-Cineole
0.50%	-	Caryophyllene oxide
0.40%	-	beta-Pinene
0.40%	-	Linalool
0.40%	-	trans-Pinocarveol
0.40%	-	Fragranyl isobutyrate
0.40%	-	trans-Fragranyl butyrate
0.40%	-	2-Methylbutyl 2-methylbutyrate
0.40%	-	Terpinen-4-yl acetate
0.30%	-	beta-Thujone
0.30%	-	p-Cymen-8-ol
0.30%	-	delta-Terpineol
0.30%	-	Fragranyl isovalerate
0.30%	-	Isoamyl acetate
0.30%	-	Isoamyl isovalerate
0.30%	-	Spathulenol
0.30%	-	Piperitol
0.30%	-	12-Methyl-13-tridecanolide
0.20%	-	Limonene
0.20%	-	Myrtenal
0.20%	-	Pinocarvone
0.20%	-	Myrtenol
0.20%	-	beta-Eudesmol
0.20%	-	trans-Carveol
0.15%	-	Cumin alcohol
0.15%	-	15-Hexadecanolide
0.10%	-	Tricyclene
0.10%	-	Terpinolene
0.10%	-	Bornyl acetate

0.10%	-	Thymol
0.10%	-	trans-Fragranyl formate
0.10%	-	tans-Verbenyl acetate
0.10%	-	Carvacrol
0.10%	-	trans-Fraaranyl caproate
0.07%	-	Cuminaldehyde
0.06%	-	Hexanal
0.05%	-	Isobutyl 2-methylbutyrate
0.05%	-	2-Pentylfuran
0.05%	-	Eugenol
0.01%	-	cis-Jasmone
93.29		TOTAL % 57 COMPOUNDS

Achillea wilhelmsii (Turkey)

BOTANICAL SPECIES

Achillea wilhelmsii C. Koch (A. santolina Auct. Mult.), fam. Asteraceae

AUTHOR

Brunke, E.-J., Hammerschmidt, F.-J., and Aboutabl, E.A.

TITLE

Volatile Constituents of Achillea Wilhelmsii C. Koch (syn. A. Santolina Auct. Mult.) from Egypt and the Turkey

PUBLICATION

In: Progress in Essential Oil Research (Proc. Intern. Symp. on Ess. Oils), E.-J. Brunke, Ed., Walter de Gruyter, Berlin (1986), 85-93

COMPOUNDS

36.10%	-	Camphor
21.40%	-	1, 8-Cineole
7.60%	-	Camphene
4.00%	-	Borneol
3.20%	-	Terpinen-4-ol
2.70%	-	alpha-Pinene
2.60%	-	Thymol
2.00%	-	para-Cymene
1.50%	-	beta-Pinene
1.50%	-	beta-Eudesmol
1.40%	-	Sabinene
1.40%	-	Artemisia alcohol
1.30%	-	alpha-Terpineol
1.20%	-	gamma-Terpinene
1.10%	-	Caryophyllene oxide

0.70%	-	alpha-Terpinene
0.70%	-	Yomogi alcohol
0.60%	-	Limonene
0.50%	-	Linalool
0.50%	-	trans-Verbenol
0.40%	-	Tricyclene
0.40%	-	Bornyl acetate
0.40%	-	delta-Terpineol
0.30%	-	Terpinolene
0.30%	-	cis-Sabinene hydrate
0.30%	-	dehydro-1, 8-Cineole
0.30%	-	Pinocarvone
0.30%	-	Spathulnol
0.30%	-	p-Metha-1,5-dien-8-ol
0.20%	-	trans-Sabinene hydrate
0.20%	-	trans-Pinocarveol
0.20%	-	trans-beta-Terpineol
0.20%	-	Myrtenol
0.20%	-	Germacrene D
0.15%	-	2-Methylbutyl 2-methylbutyrate
0.15%	-	Eugenol
0.15%	-	12-Methyl-13-tridecanolide
010%	-	Hexahydrofarnesyl acetate
0.05%	-	Isoamyl isovalerate
0.05%	-	cis-Verbenol
0.05%	-	1(7), 2-p-Menthadienol-(8)
0.05%	-	1, 5-Menthadienol-7
0.05%	-	Carvacrol
0.01%	-	15-Hexadecanolide
96.81	TOTAL %	44 COMPOUNDS

Achillea wilhelmsii (Egypt)

BOTANICAL SPECIES

Achillea wilheimsii C. Koch (A. santolina Auct. Mult.), fam. Asteraceae

AUTHOR

Brunke, E.-J., Hammerschmidt, F.-J., and AboutabI, E.A.

TITLE

Volatile Constituents of Achillea Wilheimsii C. Koch (syn. A. Santoiina Auct. Mult.) from Egypt and the Turkey

PUBLICATION

In: Progress in Essential Oil Research (Proc. Intern. Symp. on Ess. Oiis), E.-J. Brunke, Ed., Walter de Gruyter, Berlin (1986), 85-97

COMPOUNDS

25.50%	-	trans-Fragranyl acetate
15.00%	-	Camphor
13.70%	-	1, 8-Cineole
9.10%	-	Fragranol
6.90%	-	Terpinen-4-ol
3.90%	-	para-Cymene
1.90%	-	Camphene
1.50%	-	alpha-Thujone
1.10%	-	cis-Sabinene hydrate
1.00%	-	trans-Sabinene hydrate
1.00%	-	Caryophylladienols
0.90%	-	alpha-Pinene
0.60%	-	Sabinene
0.60%	-	alpha-Terpineol
0.50%	-	gamma-Terpinene

0.50%	-	Borneol
0.50%	-	Fragranyl 2-methylbutyrate
0.50%	-	dehydro-1, 8-Cineole
0.50%	-	Caryophyllene oxide
0.40%	-	beta-Pinene
0.40%	-	Linalool
0.40%	-	trans-Pinocarveol
0.40%	-	Fragranyl isobutyrate
0.40%	-	trans-Fragranyl butyrate
0.40%	-	2-Methylbutyl 2-methylbutyrate
0.40%	-	Terpinen-4-yl acetate
0.30%	-	beta-Thujone
0.30%	-	p-Cymen-8-ol
0.30%	-	delta-Terpineol
0.30%	-	Fragranyl isovalerate
0.30%	-	Isoamyl acetate
0.30%	-	Isoamyl isovalerate
0.30%	-	Spathulenol
0.30%	-	Piperitol
0.30%	-	12-Methyl-13-tridecanolide
0.20%	-	Limonene
0.20%	-	Myrtenal
0.20%	-	Pinocarvone
0.20%	-	Myrtenol
0.20%	-	beta-Eudesmol
0.20%	-	trans-Carveol
0.15%	-	Cumin alcohol
0.15%	-	15-Hexadecanolide
0.10%	-	Tricyclene
0.10%	-	Terpinolene
0.10%	-	Bornyl acetate

0.10%	-	Thymol	
0.10%	-	trans-Fragranyl formate	
0.10%	-	trans-Verbenyl acetate	
0.10%	-	Carvacrol	
010%	-	trans-Fragranyl caproate	
0.07%	-	Cuminaldehyde	
0.06%	-	Hexanal	
0.05%	-	Isobutyl 2-methylbutyrate	
0.05%	-	2-Pentylfuran	
0.05%	-	Eugenol	
0.01%	-	cis-Jasmone	
93.29		TOTAL %	57 COMPOUNDS

Yarrow (Iran)

BOTANICAL SPECIES

Achillea millefolium L. ssp. millefolium, fam. Asteraceae (Compositae)

AUTHOR

Afsharypuor, S., Asgary, S. and Lockwood, G.B.

TITLE

Volatile Constituents of Achillea millefolium L. ssp. millefolium from Iran

PUBLICATION

Flavour Fragr. J, Vol. 11, 265-267 (1996)

COMPOUNDS

22.90%	-	alpha-Bisabolol
12.40%	-	Spathulenol
5.70%	-	(Z)-Nerolidol
5.00%	-	cis-Carveol
4.00%	-	(E, E)-Farnesol
3.90%	-	Phenol
3.70%	-	trans-Carveol
2.70%	-	(Z)-beta-Farnesene
2.50%	-	cis-Sabinol
2.20%	-	alpha-Patchoulene
1.80%	-	2-Pentyl-5-propylresorcinol
1.70%	-	Campherenone
1.30%	-	Bornyl acetate
1.20%	-	beta-Himachalene
0.90%	-	Neryl acetate
0.90%	-	Geranyl acetate

0.90%	-	beta-Caryophyllene
0.90%	-	4-0xo-3,4-dihydro-2,3 diazaphenoxanthiin
0.80%	-	6,10,14-Trimethyl-2-pentadecanone
75.40		TOTAL % 19 COMPOUNDS

Yarrow

BOTANICAL SPECIES

Achillea millefolium L, fam. Asteraceae (Compositae)

AUTHOR

Falk, A.J., Bauer, L., and Bell, C.L.

TITLE

The Constituents of the Essential Oil from Achillea millefolium

PUBLICATION

Llodia, Vol. 37, 598-602 (1974)

COMPOUNDS

17.79%	-	Camphor
12.35%	-	Sabinene
9.59%	-	1, 8-Cineole
9.40%	-	alpha-Pinene
8.60%	-	iso-Artemisia ketone
7.13%	-	beta-Pinene
6.02%	-	Camphene
4.31%	-	Terpinen-4-ol
3.71%	-	gamma-Terpinene
3.69%	-	para-Cymene
2.55%	-	Borneol
2.10%	-	Bornyl acetate
1.71%	-	Limonene
1.41%	-	allo-Ocimene (unknown isomer)
1.31%	-	alpha-Terpinene
0.59%	-	Copaene (unknown isomer)
0.48%	-	Terpinolene

0.27%	-	Tricyclene
0.25%	-	Alloocimene (unknown isomer)
0.22%	-	Myrcene
0.11%	-	Cuminaldehyde
0.08%	-	delta-Cadinene
93.67		TOTAL % 22 COMPOUNDS

Yarrow (France)

BOTANICAL SPECIES

Achillea millefolium L, fam. Asteraceae (Compositae)

AUTHOR

Hachey, J.-M., Collin, G.-J., Gagnon, M.-J., Vernin, G., Fraisse, D.

TITLE

Extraction and GC/MS Analysis of the Essential Oil of Acillea millefolium L. complex (Compositae) (average conc. various samples on 2 GC-columns)

PUBLICATION

J. Ess. Oil Res., Vol. 2, 317-326, (Nov./Dec. 1990)

COMPOUNDS

13.50%	-	beta-Thujone
12.60%	-	1, 8-Cineole
10.85%	-	Camphor
7.90%	-	Sabinene
7.35%	-	beta-Pinene
5.70%	-	Terpinen-4-ol
5.20%	-	Myrcene
3.45%	-	Borneol
2.40%	-	gamma-Terpinene
2.00%	-	para-Cymene
1.95%	-	Camphene
1.70%	-	beta-Caryophyllene
1.70%	-	Chamazulene
1.55%	-	alpha-Terpineol
1.50%	-	alpha-Pinene
1.45%	-	Caryophyllene oxide

1.05%	-	Limonene
1.00%	-	Terpinolene
1.00%	-	alpha-Thujone
0.85%	-	alpha-Terpinene
0.85%	-	Bornyl acetate
0.05%	-	alpha-Phellandrene
85.60	TOTAL %	22 COMPOUNDS

Ageratum houstonianum (India)

BOTANICAL SPECIES

Ageratum houstonianum Mill., fam. Asteraceae (Compositae)

AUTHOR

Chandra, S., et al.

TITLE

Essential Oil Composition of Ageratum houstonianum Mill. from Jammu Region of India

PUBLICATION

J. Essent. Oil Res., Vol. 8, 129-134 (Mar/Apr 1996)

COMPOUNDS

43.99%	-	Precocene II
23.34%	-	Precocene I
9.18%	-	beta-Caryophyllene
2.67%	-	beta-Cubebene
2.15%	-	beta-Gurjunene
1.97%	-	Geranial
1.63%	-	Geraniol
1.32%	-	Camphene
1.31%	-	Neral
1.18%	-	Bornyl acetate
0.98%	-	(E)-beta-Farnesene
0.95%	-	Sesquiterpenes, oxygen-containing-
0.68%	-	alpha-Phellandrene
0.65%	-	Sesquiterpene hydrocarbons (unknown)
0.61%	-	Epibicyclosesquiphellandrene
0.51%	-	Geranyl acetate

0.49% - alpha-Humulene
0.33% - Limonene
0.33% - Demethoxyencecalin
0.30% - Androencecalinol
0.26% - (Z)-beta-Ocimene
0.24% - Caryophyllene oxide
0.22% - Myrcene
0.21% - Nerol
0.21% - alpha-Cubebene
0.21% - (E)-Nerolidol
0.20% - alpha-Farnesene
0.19% - alpha-Pinene
0.19% - para-Cymene
0.18% - alpha-Copaene
0.17% - 2-Carene
0.16% - (E)-beta-Ocimene
0.15% - beta-Pinene
0.14% - Eupatoriochromene
0.13% - Neryl acetate
0.13% - alpha-Muurolene
0.11% - Linalool
0.10% - Undecane
0.08% - Borneol
0.01% - gamma-Terpinene
0.01% - alpha-Ylangene
0.01% - alpha-Gurjunene
0.01% - (Z)-beta-Farnesene
0.01% - Hexadecanoic acid
0.01% - Bornyl formate
0.01% - Tetradecanoic acid
0.01% - beta-Bourbonene

0.01%	-	Germacrene B
0.01%	-	Oleic acid
0.01%	-	Octadecanoic acid
0.01%	-	2-Methylnaphthalene
0.01%	-	Dimethylnaphthalene (unknown isomer)
97.98	TOTAL %	52 COMPOUNDS

Ambrosia artemisiafolia

BOTANICAL SPECIES

Ambrosia artemisiafolia (Catinga de bode), fam. Asteraceae (Compositae)

AUTHOR

Maia, J.G.S., Ramos,L.S., Luz, A.I.R., da Silva.M.L. and Zoghbi. M.d.G.B.

TITLE

Uncommon Brazilian Essential Oils of the Labiatae and Compositae

PUBLICATION

In: Flavors and Fragr.: a World Persp., Lawrence, B.M., Mookherjee, B.D., Willis, B.J. (Eds.),Proc. of the 10th Intern. Congress of Ess. Oils, Fragr. & Flavors, Washington.DC, USA, 16-20 Nov.1986, Elsevier, Amsterdam (1988), 177-188.

COMPOUNDS

33.78%	-	beta-Himachalene
10.30%	-	gamma-Elemene
4.33%	-	delta-Elemene
4.01%	-	Bornyl acetate
3.89%	-	beta-Caryophyllene
2.38%	-	Terpinen-4-ol
1.95%	-	beta-Pinene
1.68%	-	beta-Cubebene
1.28%	-	alpha-Pinene
1.26%	-	delta-Cadinene
1.24%	-	(Z)-beta-Farnesene
0.92%	-	alpha-Humulene
0.66%	-	Copaene (unknown isomer)

0.65%	-	Limonene	
0.37%	-	Piperitone	
0.30%	-	Germacrene (unknown isomer)	
0.26%	-	trans-beta-Bergamotene	
0.24%	-	alpha-Gurjunene	
0.17%	-	gamma-Muurolene	
69.67		TOTAL %	19 COMPOUNDS

Shanqiu

BOTANICAL SPECIES

Anaphalis margaritacea (L.) Benth.et Hook. (Shanqiu), fam.Asteraceae (Comp.)

AUTHOR

Ma, J.-F, Ding, D.-S., Wang, L.-Q.

TITLE

Aroma Components of Shanqiu oil: Anaphalis margaritacea L.

PUBLICATION

In: Flavors and Fragr.: a World Persp., Lawrence, B.M., Mookerjee, B.D., Willis, B.J. (Eds.), Proc. of the 10th Intern. Congress of Ess. Oils, Fragr. & Flavors, Washington, DC, USA, 16-20 Nov. 1986, Elsevier, Amsterdam (1988), 309-316.

COMPOUNDS

22.10%	-	beta-Caryophyllene
15-98%	-	Eremophilene
8.74%	-	Aromadendrene
7.03%	-	gamma-Elemene
6.17%	-	alpha-Humulene
4.81%	-	delta-Cadinene
3.06%	-	beta-Himachalene
2.91%	-	Tricyclene
2.78%	-	ar-Curcumene
1.84%	-	2-Phenylethyl 2-methylbutyrate
1.74%	-	alpha-Fenchene
1.35%	-	Heptyl 2-methylbutyrate
0.84%	-	Gurjunene (unknown isomer)
0.50%	-	Nerolidol (unknown isomer)

0.47%	-	Bornylene
0.41%	-	alpha-Pinene
0.29%	-	Nonyl 2-methybutyrate
0.28%	-	Myrcene
0.21%	-	Terpinolene
0.21%	-	Isoheptyl 2-methylbutyrate
0.19%	-	Borneol
0.17%	-	Heptyl isobutyrate
0.11%	-	Octyl 2-methylbutyrate
0.09%	-	Geranylacetone
0.08%	-	2-Phenylethyl 3-methylbutyrate
0.06%	-	Nonanal
0.06%	-	1, 8-Cineole
0.05%	-	Pentyl 2-methylbutyrate
0.03%	-	Benzaldehyde
0.02%	-	Heptyl acetate
0.02%	-	Isoheptyl isobutyrate
0.02%	-	Isoamyl 2-methybutyrate
0.01%	-	Linalool
0.01%	-	Terpinen-4-ol
0.01%	-	Hexyl isobutyrate
82.71		TOTAL % 36 COMPOUNDS

Annual wormwood (Vietnam) 1 b

BOTANICAL SPECIES

Annua artemisia L, fam. Asteraceae (Compositae)

AUTHOR

Woerdenberg, H.J., et al.

TITLE

Volatile constituents of Artemisia annua L. (analysis of methyiene chloride extract)

PUBLICATION

Flav. Fragr. J., Vol. 8, 131-137 (1993)

COMPOUNDS

22.30%	-	Artemisinin
15.30%	-	Camphor
14.90%	-	Arteannuin B
3.10%	-	beta-Caryophyllene
2.10%	-	1, 8-Cineole
1.80%	-	Arteannuic acid
1.70%	-	Camphene
1.50%	-	alpha-Copaene
1.20%	-	(E)-beta-Farnesene
0.80%	-	Germacrene D
0.40%	-	alpha-Pinene
0.40%	-	beta-Pinene
0.40%	-	Myrcene
0.40%	-	para-Cymene
0.30%	-	alpha-Guaiene
0.30%	-	Cadinol (unknown structure)
0.20%	-	Borneol

0.20%	-	cis-Chrysanthenyl acetate
0.20%	-	trans-Chrysantenyl acetate
0.10%	-	trans-Sabinene hydrate
0.10%	-	beta-Elemene
0.05%	-	alpna-Thujene
0.05%	-	Sabinene
0.05%	-	cis-Sabinene hydrate
0.05%	-	cis-Chrysanthenol
67.90	TOTAL %	25 COMPOUNDS

Roman chamomile (India)

BOTANICAL SPECIES

Anthemis nobilis L, fam. Asteraceae (Compositae)

AUTHOR

Shaath, N.A., Dedeian-Johnson, S., and Griffin, P.M.

TITLE

The Analysis of Chamomile Roman

PUBLICATION

In: Proceedings 11th Intern. Congress of Essential Oils, Fragrances and Flavours, 12-16 Nov., 1989, New Delhi, India, Vol. 4, 207-213

COMPOUNDS

20.97%	-	3-Methylpentyl isovalerate
15.83%	-	Methallyl angelate
11.88%	-	3-Methylpentyl isobutyrate
7.83%	-	2-Methylbutyl angelate
4.79%	-	trans-Pinocarveol
4.10%	-	Isoamyl angelate
3.44%	-	isobutyl angelate
2.96%	-	alpha-Pinene
2.62%	-	3-Methylpentyl methacrylate
2.22%	-	Isoamyl isobutyrate
1.30%	-	3-Methylpentyl 2-methylbutyrate
1.16%	-	2-Melhylbutyl methacrylate
1.00%	-	1-Nonen-3-ol
0.83%	-	Propyl angelate
0.75%	-	Sesquiterpene hydrocarbons (unknown)
0.70%	-	Isobutyl isobutyrate

0.69% - Isoprenyl angelate
0.66% - 3-Methylpentyl propionate
0.62% - 2-Methylbutyl acetate
0.55% - Camphene
0.51% - Isoamyl methacrylate
0.38% - Myrtenol
0.35% - Butyl angelate
0.31% - beta-Pinene
0.30% - (E)-beta-Farnesene
0.28% - 3-Methylpentanol
0.23% - Isoborneol
0.22% - beta-Selinene
0.22% - 2-Methylbutyl 2-menthylbutyrate
0.18% - Isoamyl 2-menthylbutyrate
0.16% - Prenyl isobutyrate
0.15% - Methallyl tiglate
0.13% - Prenyl angelate
0.12% - Isoamyl acetate
0.12% - Ethyl angelate
0.11% - beta-Bisabolene
0.11% - Germacrene D
0.10% - Myrcene
0.09% - Limonene
0.08% - 1, 8-Cineole
0.08% - 3-Methylbutyl propionate
0.07% - 2-Methylbutyl tiglate
0.06% - Prenyl acetate
0.06% - Propyl isobutyrate
0.05% - 2-Phenylethyl isobutyrate
0.05% - Isoprenyl tiglate
0.05% - Geranyl isobutyrate

0.05%	-	(E, E)-alpha-Farnesene
0.04%	-	Sabinene
0.04%	-	Ethyl 2-methylbutyrate
0.04%	-	Butyl methacrylate
0.03%	-	Benzaldehyde
0.03%	-	Verbenone
0.03%	-	Isobutyl tiglate
0.03%	-	isoamyl tiglate
0.02%	-	2-Methylbutanol
0.02%	-	3-Methylbutanol
0.01%	-	para-Cymene
0.01%	-	Terpinen-4-ol
0.01%	-	(Z) 3-Hexenyl acetate
0.01%	-	Ethyl isobutyrate
0.01%	-	Isobutyl acetate
89.85	TOTAL %	62 COMPOUNDS

Roman chamomile (Italy) 1

BOTANICAL SPECIES

Anthemis nobilis L, fam. Asteraceae (Compositae)

AUTHOR

Nano, G.M., Sacco, T., and Frattini, C.

TITLE

Botanical and chemical research on Anthemis nobilis L. and some of its cultivars

PUBLICATION

Essenze Deriv.Agrum., Vol. 93, 107-114 (1973); Paper No. 114, 6th International Essential Oil Congress, San Francisco (1974)

COMPOUNDS

12.00%	-	1, 8-Cineole
12.00%	-	2-Methylbutyl 2-methylbutyrate
12.00%	-	Isobutyl angelate
12.00%	-	2-Methylbutyl 2-methylpropionate
5.00%	-	alpha-Pinene
5.00%	-	Sabinene
5.00%	-	beta-Pinene
5.00%	-	beta-Caryophyllene
5.00%	-	Myrtenal
5.00%	-	Hexyl acetate
5.00%	-	Butyl angelate
5.00%	-	2-Methylbutyl butyrate
5.00%	-	2-Methylbutyl 3-methylbutyrate
5.00%	-	Propyl angelate
0.25%	-	Camphene
0.25%	-	Myrcene

0.25%	-	para-Cymene	
0.25%	-	gamma-Terpinene	
0.25%	-	delta-Cadinene	
0.25%	-	Copaene (unknown isomer)	
0.25%	-	alpha, p-Dimethylstyrene	
0.25%	-	beta-Copaene	
100.00		TOTAL %	22 COMPOUNDS

Roman chamomile (Italy) 3

BOTANICAL SPECIES

Anthemis nobilis L, fam. Asteraceae (Compositae)

AUTHOR

Chialva, F., Gabri, G., Liddie, P.A.P., and Ulian, F.

TITLE

Qualitative Evaluation of Aromatic Herbs by Direct Headspace GC Analysis. Applications of the Method and Comparison with the Trad. Analysis of E.O.

PUBLICATION

Journal of HRC & CC, Vol. 5, April 1982, 182-188

COMPOUNDS

36.00%	-	Isobutyl angelate
17.90%	-	Isoamyl angelate
7.40%	-	2-Methyl-2-propy! angelate
3.90%	-	Hexyl butyrate
3.70%	-	Isobutyl isobutyrate
2.80%	-	Isoamyl 2-methylbutyrate
2.70%	-	2-Methylbutyl 2-methylbutyrate
2.60%	-	Isoamyl butyrate
1.60%	-	alpha-Pinene
1.10%	-	Propyl angelate
0.90%	-	Butyl angelate
0.40%	-	Camphene
0.20%	-	beta-Pinene
0.20%	-	Limonene
81.40	TOTAL %	14 COMPOUNDS

Roman chamomile (Italy) 2 (headspace)

BOTANICAL SPECIES

Anthemis nobilis L, fam. Asteraceae (Compositae)

AUTHOR

Chiaiva, F., Gabri, G., Liddie, P.A.P., and Uiian, F.

TITLE

Qualitative Evaluation of Aromatic Herbs by Direct Headspace GC Analysis. Applications of the Method and Comparison with the Trad. Analysis of E.O.

PUBLICATION

Journal of HRC & CC, Vol. 5, April 1982, 182-188

COMPOUNDS

36.50%	-	Isobutyl angelate
12.70%	-	Isobutyl isobutyrate
8.40%	-	Isoamyl angelate
5.80%	-	2-Methyl-2-propyl angelate
3.70%	-	alpha-Pinene
3.40%	-	Isoamyl butyrate
1.40%	-	Hexyl butyrate
1.10%	-	Camphene
1.10%	-	Propyl angelate
0.80%	-	Isobutyl 2-methylbutyrate
0.80%	-	Isoamyl 2-methylbutyrate
0.20%	-	Butyl angelate
0.05%	-	beta-Pinene
0.05%	-	Limonene
0.05%	-	2-Methylbutyl 2-methylbutyrate
76.05	TOTAL %	15 COMPOUNDS

Roman chamomile (Italy) 5

BOTANICAL SPECIES

Anthemis nobilis L., fam. Asteraceae (Compositae)

AUTHOR

Zani, F., et al.

TITLE

Studies on the genotoxic properties of essential oils with Bacillus subtilis recassay and salmonella/mircosome reversion assay

PUBLICATION

Planta med. Vol. 57, 237-241 (1991)

COMPOUNDS

34.90%	-	Butyl angelate
15.85%	-	Isoamyl angelate
5.04%	-	Borneol
4.12%	-	alpha-Thujene
2.75%	-	delta-3-Carene
1.61%	-	alpha-Pinene
1.07%	-	beta-Pinene
0.72%	-	Myrcene
0.54%	-	Camphene
0.40%	-	alpha-Thujone
0.30%	-	Carvacrol
67.30	TOTAL %	11 COMPOUNDS

Roman chamomile (Italy) 4

BOTANICAL SPECIES

Anthemis nobilis L, fam. Asteraceae (Compositae)

AUTHOR

Srinivas, S.R.

TITLE

Atlas of Essential Oils

PUBLICATION

see title: S.R. Srinivas, Bronx, NY (1986)

COMPOUNDS

37.41%	-	Isobutyl angelate
20.33%	-	3-Methylpentyl angelate
10.78%	-	Isoamyl angelate
5.00%	-	Camphene
3.98%	-	alpha-Terpinene
3.47%	-	Chamazulene
3.00%	-	Anthemol
2.80%	-	gamma-Terpinene
2.10%	-	Myrcene
1.61%	-	alpha-Pinene
0.71%	-	beta-Pinene
91.19	TOTAL %	11 COMPOUNDS

Roman chamomile (Egypt)

BOTANICAL SPECIES

Anthemis nobilis L., fam. Asteraceae (Compositae)

AUTHOR

Srinivas, S.R.

TITLE

Atlas of Essential Oils

PUBLICATION

see title, S.R. Srinivas, Bronx, N.Y. (1986)

COMPOUNDS

33.94%	-	Isobutyl angelate
18.32%	-	3-Methylpentyl angelate
8.39%	-	Isoamyl angelate
4.52%	-	alpha-Pinene
3.81%	-	alpha-Terpinene
3.22%	-	gamma-Terpinene
2.07%	-	Chamazulene
1.45%	-	Anthemol
1.42%	-	Myrcene
0.58%	-	beta-Pinene
77.72	TOTAL %	10 COMPOUNDS

Roman chamomile (England)

BOTANICAL SPECIES

Anthemis nobilis L., fam. Asteraceae (Compositae)

AUTHOR

Srinivas, S.R.

TITLE

Atlas of Essential Oils

PUBLICATION

See title: S.R. Srinivas, Bronx, NY (1986)

COMPOUNDS

20.52%	-	Isobutyl butyrate
17.38%	-	Isoamyl angelate
16.22%	-	3-Methylpentyl angelate
13.01%	-	Isobutyl angelate
4.51%	-	alpha-Terpinene
4.39%	-	Chamazulene
3.85%	-	Terpinolene
3.22%	-	Anthemol
2.86%	-	gamma-Terpinene
2.01%	-	para-Cymene
1.60%	-	beta-Pinene
1.58%	-	alpha-Pinene
1.38%	-	beta-Phellandrene
1.37%	-	Camphene
0.46%	-	p-Cymen-8-ol
94.36	TOTAL %	15 COMPOUNDS

Roman chamomile (Japan)

BOTANICAL SPECIES

Anthemis nobilis L, fam. Asteraceae (Compositae)

AUTHOR

Hasebe, A. and Oomura, T.

TITLE

The Constituents of the essential oils from Anthemis nobilis L. (Roman chamomile) (only main constituents; 57 trace constituents)

PUBLICATION

Koryo (161), 93-101 (1989)

COMPOUNDS

35.92%	-	Isobutyl angelate
15.29%	-	2-Melhylbutyl angelate
8.71%	-	Methallyl angelate
4.91%	-	Isobutyl isobutyrate
4.34%	-	Isoamyl angelate
3.59%	-	Pinocarvone
3.05%	-	2-Methylbutyl 2-methyipropionate
2.86%	-	trans-Pinocarveol
2.15%	-	alpha-Pinene
1.62%	-	Isobutyl methacrylate
1.33%	-	Propyl angelate
1.04%	-	Isobutyl 2-metnylbutyrate
0.98%	-	Isoamyl methacrylate
0.77%	-	(E)-2-Methyl-2-butenyl angelate
0.76%	-	Butyl angelate
0.72%	-	Camphene

0.52%	-	2-Hydroxy-2-methyl-3-butenyl angelate
0.46%	-	Myrtenal
0.44%	-	Isoamyl tiglate
0.42%	-	Isobutyl 3-hydroxy-2-methylidene-butyrate
0.35%	-	Isoamyl acetate
0.34%	-	Isobutyl tiglate
0.34%	-	beta-Methallyl isobutyrate
0.34%	-	beta-Methallyl methacrylate
0.33%	-	(E)-2-Methyl-2-butenyl acetate
0.27%	-	Sabinene
0.27%	-	Myrtenol
0.27%	-	Isoamyl 3-hydroxy—methylidene-butyrate
0.25%	-	3-Methylpentyl angelate
0.22%	-	Methallyl tiglate
0.21%	-	alpha-Terpineol
0.20%	-	beta-Pinene
0.18%	-	Geranyl acetate
0.18%	-	2-Methylbutyl tiglate
0.14%	-	6, 10, 14-Trimethyl-2-pentadecanone
0.12%	-	Pinocamphone
0.12%	-	Butyl tiglate
0.12%	-	Amyl angelate
0.11%	-	beta-Terpineol
0.11%	-	Propyl isobutyrate
0.10%	-	Benzyl acetate
0.10%	-	3-Hydroxy-2-methyiidenebutyl angelate
94.55		TOTAL % 42 COMPOUNDS

Artemisia abaensis (China)

BOTANICAL SPECIES

Artemisia abaensis Y.R. Ling et S.Y. Zhao, fam. Asteraceae (Compositae)

AUTHOR

Liangfeng Zhu, Li Yonghua, Li Baoling, Lu Biyao & Xia Nianhe

TITLE

Aromatic Plants and Essential Constituents p. 272

PUBLICATION

South China Institute of Botany, Chinese Academy of Sciences, Hai Feng Publishing Co., Chinese National Node for APINMAP, distributed by Peace Book Co. Ltd., Hong Kong (1993)

COMPOUNDS

15.48%	-	Camphor
8.47%	-	1, 8-Cineole
5.93%	-	Artemisia ketone
5.11%	-	3-Hexenyl butyrate
3.14%	-	Borneol
2.38%	-	Cadinol (unknown structure)
2.18%	-	beta-Eudesmol
1.40%	-	Artemisiatriene
1.28%	-	2-Methyl-6-methylene-1,7-octadien-3-one
1.26%	-	Terpinen-4-ol
1.00%	-	para-Cymene
1.00%	-	beta-Selinene
0.87%	-	Sabinene
0.83%	-	alpha-Thujone
0.69%	-	4-Methyl-3-pentenal

0.62%	-	Indole	
0.55%	-	1-Nonen-3-ol	
0.55%	-	alpha-Selinol	
0.53%	-	gamma-Cadinene	
0.47%	-	alpha-Curcumene	
0.42%	-	Benzaldehyde	
0.39%	-	Hexanal	
0.39%	-	Phenylacetaldehyde	
0.38%	-	cis-Sabinyl acetate	
0.31%	-	alpha-Terpineol	
0.29%	-	beta-Farnesene	
0.24%	-	7-Octen-4-ol	
0.21%	-	Methyl eugenol	
0.20%	-	6-Methyl-5-hepten-2-One	
0.19%	-	Jasmone	
0.12%	-	3, 6, 6-Trimethyl-2-norpinanol	
56.88		TOTAL %	31 COMPOUNDS

Artemisia abrotanum (Italy)

BOTANICAL SPECIES

Artemisia abrotanum L, fam. Asteraceae (Compositae)

AUTHOR

Mucciarelli, M., Caramiello, R., Maffei, M., and Chialva, F.

TITLE

Essential Oils from Some Artemisia Species Growing Spontaneously in North-West Italy (0.01 % = trace)

PUBLICATION

Flavour Fragr. J., Vol. 10, 25-32 (1995)

COMPOUNDS

34.70%	-	1, 8-Cineole
18.40%	-	Bisabolol oxide (unknown isomer)
16.00%	-	Ascaridole
7.90%	-	para-Cymene
4.20%	-	(E)-Nerolidol
4.00%	-	Spathulenol
3.30%	-	Bornyl acetate
3.10%	-	Carvacrol
2.20%	-	Terpinen-4-ol
1.80%	-	Pinocarvone
1.00%	-	Myrtenol
0.70%	-	alpha-Terpineol
0.60%	-	alpha-Phellandrene
0.60%	-	alpha-Terpinene
0.50%	-	gamma-Terpinene
0.40%	-	alpha-Thujone
0.40%	-	beta-Thujone

0.30% - Limonene
0.01% - alpha-Thujene
0.01% - alpha-Pinene
0.01% - Camphene
0.01% - Sabinene
0.01% - beta-Pinene
0.01% - Myrcene
0.01% - Terpinolene
0.01% - Linalool
0.01% - Borneol
0.01% - Camphor
0.01% - Carvone
0.01% - beta-Caryophyllene
0.01% - alpha-Copaene
0.01% - Myrtenal
0.01% - trans-Pinocarveol
0.01% - dehydro-1, 8-Cineole
0.01% - Yomogi alcohol
0.01% - Artemisia alcohol
0.01% - cis-Verbenol
0.01% - Caryophyllene oxide
0.01% - Sabinene hydrate
0.01% - Cubenol
0.01% - alpha-Cadinol
0.01% - Verbenone
0.01% - alpha-Fenchene
0.01% - trans-Carveol
0.01% - alpha-Bisabolol
0.01% - Cuminaldehyde
0.01% - Artemisia ketone
0.01% - Artemisyl acetate

0.01%	-	cis-Chrysanthenyl acetate
0.01%	-	Linalool oxides (cis/trans) (unknown isomers)
0.01%	-	beta-Damascenone
0.01%	-	Camphenilone
0.01%	-	delta-Selinene
0.01%	-	Isopinocamphone
0.01%	-	trans-alpha-Bergamotol
0.01%	-	Sabinyl acetate
0.01%	-	trans-Chrysantenyl acetate
0.01%	-	cis-Ocimene epoxide
0.01%	-	cis-2-Thujenol-4
0.01%	-	Nojigiku alcohol
100.52		TOTAL % . 60 COMPOUNDS

Wormwood (Mugwort) (India)

BOTANICAL SPECIES

Artemisia absinthum L., fam. Asteraceae (Compositae)

AUTHOR

Kaul, V.K., Nigam, S.S., and Banerjee, A.K.

TITLE

Thin-layer and gas chromatographic studies of the essential oil of Artemisia absinthum L.

PUBLICATION

Indian Perf., Vol. 23, 1-7 (1979)

COMPOUNDS

22.00%	-	alpha-Thujone
20.23%	-	Thujyl alcohol
11.50%	-	Thujyl acetate
10.54%	-	beta-Phellandrene
6.94%	-	alpha-Himachalene
5.41%	-	beta-Caryophyllene
2.57%	-	Anisaldenyde
2.45%	-	alpha-Terpineol
1.42%	-	Geraniol
1.28%	-	Caryophyllene oxide
1.25%	-	alpha-Cadinene
1.22%	-	Elemol
1.20%	-	Methyl heptenone (unknown structure)
0.97%	-	1, 8-Cineole
0.96%	-	alpha-Pinene
0.25%	-	para-Cymene
0.15%	-	Camphene
0.10%	-	alpha-Thujene
90.44	TOTAL %	18 COMPOUNDS

Wormwood (Mugwort) (Spain)

BOTANICAL SPECIES

Artemisia absinthum L., fam. Asteraceae (Compositae)

AUTHOR

de Gavina Mugica, M., and Ochoa, J.T.

TITLE

Aceite esencial de Artemisia absinthum L.

PUBLICATION

In: Contribucion ai estudio de Ios aceites esenciales Espanoles; 11. Aceites esenciales de la provincia de Guadalajara. Instituto Nacional Investigaciones Agrarias Minist. Agric. Madrid (1974)

COMPOUNDS

63.30%	-	Thujone (unknown isomer)
6.50%	-	Camphor
6.00%	-	Citronellal
3.90%	-	para-Cymene
2.00%	-	1, 8-Cineole
1.90%	-	Limonene
1.20%	-	Camphnene
1.20%	-	Carvotanacetone
1 .00%	-	alpha-Pinene
1.00%	-	Thujane
0.85%	-	Sabinene
0.85%	-	beta-Pinene
0.60%	-	Myrcene
0.40%	-	Geranial
0.20%	-	gamma-Terpinene
0.20%	-	Perillaldehyde

0.20%	-	Benzyl benzoate	
0.15%	-	Carvone	
0.15%	-	cis-Sabinol	
0.10%	-	alpha-Phellandrene	
0.10%	-	Borneol	
0.10%	-	alpha-Terpineol	
0.10%	-	Neral	
0.10%	-	Methyl chavicol	
0.10%	-	Thujyl alcohol	
0.05%	-	alpha-Thujene	
0.05%	-	Eugenol	
92.30		TOTAL%	27 COMPOUNDS

Wormwood (Mugwort)

BOTANICAL SPECIES

Artemisia absinthum L., fam. Asteraceae (Compositae)

AUTHOR

Chialva, F., Gabri, G., Liddle, P.A.P., and Ulian, F.

TITLE

Qualitative Evaluation of Aromatic Herbs by Direct Headspace GC Analysis. Applications of the Method and Comparison with the Trad. Analysis of E.O.

PUBLICATION

Journal of HRC & CC, Vol. 5, April 1982, 182-188

COMPOUNDS

16.70%	-	cis-Epoxycymene
6.00%	-	Linalool
4.40%	-	Chrysanthenyl acetate
3.20%	-	Neryl/geranyl 2-methylbutyrate
3.10%	-	Geraniol
2.70%	-	beta-Thujone
2.50%	-	Camphor
2.20%	-	trans-Epoxycymene
2.10%	-	Neryl isovalerate
1.60%	-	beta-Caryophyllene
1.20%	-	Nerol
1.20%	-	Chamazulene
1.00%	-	alpha-Bisabolol
0.70%	-	beta-Bourbonene
0.40%	-	Eugenol
0.40%	-	alpha-Cubebene

0.20%	-	beta-Pinene	
0.20%	-	Myrcene	
0.10%	-	alpha-Pinene	
0.10%	-	Camphene	
0.05%	-	para-Cymene	
0.05%	-	Limonene	
0.05%	-	gamma-Terpinene	
0.05%	-	1, 8-Cineole	
50.20		TOTAL %	24 COMPOUNDS

Wormwood (Mugwort), headspace

BOTANICAL SPECIES

Artemisia absinthum L., fam. Asteraceae (Compositae)

AUTHOR

Chialva, F., Gabri, G., Liddie, P.A.P., and Ulian, F.

TITLE

Qualitative Evaluation of Aromatic Herbs by Direct Headspace GC Analysis. Applications of the Method and Comparison with the Trad. Analysis of E.O.

PUBLICATION

Journal of HRC & CC, Vol. 5, April 1982, 182-188

COMPOUNDS

10.60%	-	Linalool	
10.30%	-	cis-Epoxycymene	
6.00%	-	Terpinen-4-ol	
2.60%	-	alpha-Pinene	
2.60%	-	beta-Pinene	
2.30%	-	Myrcene	
2.00%	-	beta-Thujone	
1.50%	-	Camphor	
0.80%	-	Camphene	
0.70%	-	trans-Epoxycymene	
0.60%	-	alpha-Phellandrene	
0.60%	-	Chrysanthenyl acetate	
0.05%	-	para-Cymene	
0.05%	-	Limonene	
0.05%	-	gamma-Terpinene	
0.05%	-	1, 8-Cineole	
40.80		TOTAL %	16 COMPOUNDS

Wormwood (Mugwort) (Germany)

BOTANICAL SPECIES

Artemisia absinthum L, fam. Asteraceae (Compositae)

AUTHOR

Vostrowsky, O., Brosche, T., Ihm, H., Zintl, R., and Knobloch, K.

TITLE

Ueber die Komponenten des aetherischen Oels aus Artemisia absinthum L.

PUBLICATION

Z. Naturforsch., Vol. 36c, 369-377 (1981)

COMPOUNDS

46.44%	-	beta-Thujone
25.00%	-	Sabinyl acetate
3.21%	-	trans-Sabinol
2.78%	-	Lavandulyl acetate
2.76%	-	alpha-Thujone
2.71%	-	Sabinene
1.43%	-	Geranyl propionate
1.15%	-	Myrcene
0.71%	-	1, 8-Cineole
0.70%	-	(Z)-3-Hexenol
0.50%	-	Lavandulol
0.44%	-	Terpinen-4-ol
0.43%	-	alpha-Pinene
0.34%	-	para-Cymene
0.33%	-	Geranyl acetate
0.32%	-	gamma-Cadinene

0.20%	-	Camphene
0.20%	-	1-Octene
0.18%	-	alpha-Copaene
0.16%	-	alpha-Terpineol
0.15%	-	alpha-Phellandrene
0.14%	-	gamma-Terpinene
0.13%	-	Xylenes
0.12%	-	alpha-Humulene
0.10%	-	cis-Sabinyl acetate
0.09%	-	Pulegone
0.07%	-	Linalool
0.06%	-	beta-Pinene
0.06%	-	Neryl acetate
0.06%	-	beta-Caryophyllene
0.06%	-	trans-Sabiene hydrate
0.06%	-	1-Nonanol
0.05%	-	alpha-Thujene
0.05%	-	Terpinolene
0.05%	-	cis-Piperitol
0.05%	-	trans-Piperitol
0.05%	-	Thujyl alcohol
0.04%	-	Borneol
0.04%	-	cis-Piperityl acetate
0.02%	-	(E)-beta-Ocimene
0.01%	-	alpha-Terpinene
0.01%	-	Nerol
0.01%	-	Carvone
0.01%	-	trans-Piperityl acetate

91.48	TOTAL %	44 COMPOUNDS

Wormwood (Mugwort) (U.S.A.) 1

BOTANICAL SPECIES

Artemisia absinthum L., fam. Asteraceae (Compositae)

AUTHOR

Lawrence, B.M.

TITLE

Chemical Composition of some Wormwood oils produced in North America

PUBLICATION

Pert. Flav., Vol. 17, 42 (March/April 1992)

COMPOUNDS

40.00%	-	cis-Sabinyl acetate
35.00%	-	bela-Thujone
6.32%	-	Sabinene
3.71%	-	Linalool
2.41%	-	beta-Caryophyllene
1.90%	-	1, 8-Cineole
0.96%	-	Caryophyllene oxide
0.87%	-	alpha-Thujone
0.48%	-	Germacrene D
0.46%	-	alpha-Pinene
0.43%	-	Myrcene
0.29%	-	cis-Sabinol
0.27%	-	para-Cymene
0.19%	-	beta-Pinene
0.13%	-	Camphor
0.11%	-	gamma-Terpinene
0.10%	-	beta-Phellandrene

0.09%	-	Limonene
0.07%	-	cis-Ocimene epoxide
0.06%	-	alpha-Terpinene
0.05%	-	alpha-Phellandrene
0.03%	-	Terpinolene
0.02%	-	Camphene
0.01%	-	(Z)-beta-Ocimene
0.01%	-	(E)-beta-0cimene
93.97	TOTAL %	25 COMPOUNDS

Wormwood (Mugwort) (Italy) 1

BOTANICAL SPECIES

Artemisia absinthum L., fam. Asteraceae (Compositae)

AUTHOR

Chialva, F., Liddle, P.A.P., and Doglia, G.

TITLE

Chemotaxonomy of Wormwood (Artemisia absinthum L.) I. Composition of the essential oil of several chemotypes (Epoxy-ocimene: average 10 samples)

PUBLICATION

Z. Lebensmitt. Unters. Forsch., Vol. 176, 363-366 (1983)

COMPOUNDS

40.00%	-	cis-Ocimene epoxide
5.50%	-	Chrysanthendiol
4-00%	-	Chrysanthenyl acetate
3.50%	-	cis-Sabinyl acetate
2.00%	-	Sabinene
2.00%	-	Camphor
2.00%	-	beta-Thujone
2.00%	-	alpha-Bisabolol
2.00%	-	trans-Ocimene epoxide
2.00%	-	Neryl isovalerate
2.00%	-	Neryl butyrate
1.50%	-	Myrcene
1.50%	-	beta-Caryophyllene
1.50%	-	Germacrene D
1.50%	-	Sabinol
1.30%	-	Nerol

1.08%	-	alpha-Pinene
1.00%	-	Linalool
1.00%	-	Geranyl acetate
1.00%	-	beta-Ocimene
1.00%	-	Neryl isobutyrate
0.50%	-	Spathulenol
0.50%	-	beta-Curcumene
0.20%	-	Limonene
0.20%	-	1, 8-Cineole
0.20%	-	Neryl acetate
0.20%	-	Geranyl butyrate
0.15%	-	alpha-Thujone
0.15%	-	Geranyl isobutyrate
0.10%	-	para-Cymene
0.10%	-	Gerayl 3-methylbutyrate
81.68	TOTAL%	31 COMPOUNDS

Wormwood (Mugwort) (U.S.A.) 2

BOTANICAL SPECIES

Artemisia absinthum L, fam. Asteraceae (Compositae)

AUTHOR

Tucker, A.O., M.J. Maciarello & G. Sturtz

TITLE

The Essential Oils of Artemisia 'Powis Castle' and Its Putative Parents, A. absinthium and A. arborescens (commercial sample)

PUBLICATION

J. Essent. Oil Res., Vol. 5, 239-242 (May/Jun 1993)

COMPOUNDS

33.11%	-	beta-Thujone
32.75%	-	cis-Sabinyl acetate
3.42%	-	alpha-Thujone
2.91%	-	Sabinene
2.70%	-	cis-Sabinol
2.08%	-	Geranyl propionate
1.81%	-	Lavandulyl acetate
1.74%	-	Linalool
1.72%	-	Germacrene D
1.44%	-	beta-Caryophyllene
1.44%	-	Neryl isobutyrate
1.32%	-	Myrcene
0.97%	-	beta-Selinene
0.85%	-	cis-Ocimene epoxide
0.71%	-	Lavandulol
0.69%	-	alpha-Pinene
0.62%	-	1, 8-Cineole

0.41%	-	gamma-Terpinene
0.39%	-	(Z)-3-Hexenol
0.37%	-	Nerol
0.35%	-	alpha-Phellandrene
0.28%	-	para-Cymene
0.24%	-	cis-Salvene
0.21%	-	Limonene
0.19%	-	beta-Pinene
0.18%	-	alpha-Fenchene
0.16%	-	alpha-Terpinene
0.14%	-	Geraniol
0.11%	-	Chamazulene
0.05%	-	Terpinolene
93.36	TOTAL%	30 COMPOUNDS

Wormwood (Mugwort) (U.S.A.) 3

BOTANICAL SPECIES

Artemisia absinthum L., fam. Asteraceae (Compositae)

AUTHOR

Tucker, A.O., M.J. Maciarello & G. Sturtz

TITLE

The Essential Oils of Artemisia 'Powis Castie' and Its Putative Patents, A. absinthium and A. arborescens (analyses of 3 lab-dist. samples)

PUBLICATION

J. Essent. Oil Res, Vol. 5, 239-242 (May/Jun 1993)

COMPOUNDS

29.85%	-	Sabinene
29.83%	-	Myrcene
19.02%	-	alpha-Phellandrene
2.12%	-	para-Cymene
1.17%	-	Neryl acetate
0.96%	-	(Z)-3-Hexenyl acetate
0.40%	-	alpha-Fenchene
0.36%	-	gamma-Terpinene
0.23%	-	alpha-Pinene
0.14%	-	beta-Phellandrene
0.05%	-	Limonene
0.04%	-	beta-Pinene
0.04%	-	alpha-Terpinene
84.21	TOTAL %	13 COMPOUNDS

Wormwood (Mugwort) (Italy) 2

BOTANICAL SPECIES

Artemisia absinthum L, fam. Asteraceae (Compositae)

AUTHOR

Mucciarelli, M., Caramiello, R., Maffei, M., and Chialva, F.

TITLE

Essential Oils from Some Artemisia Species Growing Spontaneously in North-West Italy (0.01% = trace)

PUBLICATION

Flavour Fragr. J., Vol. 10, 25-32 (1995)

COMPOUNDS

24.80%	-	cis-Ocimene epoxide
21.60%	-	trans-Chrysantenyl acetate
17.10%	-	Camphor
10.00%	-	Caryophyllene oxide
7.90%	-	Spathulenol
4.50%	-	Bisabolol oxide (unknown isomer)
2.50%	-	Borneol
1.70%	-	Linalool
1.40%	-	1, 8-Cineole
1.40%	-	beta-Caryophyllene
1.30%	-	alpha-Pinene
1.30%	-	beta-Thujone
1.30%	-	Artemisyl acetate
1.20%	-	Camphene
1.10%	-	alpha-Fenchene
1.00%	-	para-Cymene
0.01%	-	alpha-Thujene

0.01% - Sabinene
0.01% - beta-Pinene
0.01% - Myrcene
0.01% - alpha-Phellandrene
0.01% - alpha-Terpinene
0.01% - Limonene
0.01% - gamma-Terpinene
0.01% - Terpinolene
0.01% - Terpinen-4-ol
0.01% - alpha-Terpineol
0.01% - Carvone
0.01% - Bornyl acetate
0.01% - alpha-Copaene
0.01% - alpha-Thujone
0.01% - Myrtenal
0.01% - dehydro-1, 8-Cineole
0.01% - Yomogi alcohol
0.01% - Artemisia alcohol
0.01% - Pinocarvone
0.01% - trans-Verbenol
0.01% - Myrtenol
0.01% - Carvacrol
0.01% - Sabinene hydrate
0.01% - (E)-Nerolidol
0.01% - alpha-Cadinol
0.01% - Pinocarveol
0.01% - Verbenone
0.01% - trans-Carveol
0.01% - alpha-Bisabolol
0.01% - Cuminaldehyde
0.01% - Artemisia ketone

0.01%	-	cis-Chrysanthenyl acetate
0.01%	-	Linalool oxides (cis/trans) (unknown isomers)
0.01%	-	beta-Damascenone
0.01%	-	Ascaridole
0.01%	-	gamma-Selinene
0.01%	-	1-epi-Cubenol
0.01%	-	Camphenllone
0.01%	-	Isopinocamphone
0.01%	-	trans-alpha-Bergamotol
0.01%	-	Sabinyl acetate
0.01%	-	cis-2-Thujenol-4
0.01%	-	Nojigiku alcohol
100.54	TOTAL %	60 COMPOUNDS

Wormwood (Mugwort) (U.S.A.) 4

BOTANICAL SPECIES

Artemisia absinthum L., var. 'Powis Castle', fam. Asteraceae (Compositae)

AUTHOR

Tucker, A.O., M.J. Maciarello & G. Sturtz

TITLE

The Essential Oils of Artemisia 'Powis Castle' and Its Putative Parents, A. absinthium and A. arborescens (analysis of field-distilled oil)

PUBLICATION

J. Essent. Oil Res., Vol. 5, 239-242 (May/Jun 1993)

COMPOUNDS

38.36%	-	beta-Thujone
25.80%	-	cis-Ocimene epoxide
6.03%	-	(Z)-beta-Ocimene
3.61%	-	Chamazulene
3.48%	-	Germacrene D
2.39%	-	Sabinene
2.36%	-	alpha-Thujone
2.29%	-	Camphor
1.85%	-	beta-Caryophyllene
1.77%	-	Myrcene
1.02%	-	Linalool
0.98%	-	alpha-Pinene
0.74%	-	trans-Ocimene epoxide
0.55%	-	Neryl isobutyrate
0.50%	-	(E)-beta-Ocimene
0.42%	-	Camphene

0.42%	-	1, 8-Cineole	
0.33%	-	Limonene	
0.30%	-	Geranyl propionate	
0.18%	-	beta-Pinene	
0.15%	-	alpha-Terpinene	
0.06%	-	Terpinolene	
93.59		TOTAL %	22 COMPOUNDS

Wormwood (Mugwort) (U.S.A.) 5

BOTANICAL SPECIES

Artemisia absinthum L., var. 'Powis Castle", fam. Asteraceae (Compositae)

AUTHOR

Tucker, A.O., M.J. Maciarello & G. Sturtz

TITLE

The Essential Oils of Artemisia 'Powis Castle' and its Putative Parents, A. absinthium and A. arborescens (average of 3 lab-distilled samples)

PUBLICATION

J. Essent. Oil Res., Vol. 5, 239-242 (May/Jun 1993)

COMPOUNDS

41.21%	-	beta-Thujone
24.76%	-	cis-Ocimene epoxide
7.36%	-	(Z)-beta-Ocimene
2.99%	-	Camphor
2.73%	-	Sabinene
2.27%	-	alpha-Thujone
2.22%	-	Chamazulene
1.87%	-	Germacrene D
1.34%	-	Myrcene
1.30%	-	Linalool
1.20%	-	alpha-Pinene
1.18%	-	beta-Caryophyllene
0.52%	-	trans-Ocimene epoxide
0.52%	-	(E)-beta-Ocimene
0.38%	-	Camphene
0.25%	-	Limonene

0.17%	-	beta-Pinene
0.14%	-	alpha-Terpinene
0.07%	-	1, 8-Cineole
0.05%	-	Geranyl propionate
0.02%	-	Terpinolene
92.65	TOTAL %	21 COMPOUNDS

Lanyana (Oregon-USA)

BOTANICAL SPECIES

Artemisia afra Jacq., fam. Asteraceae (Compositae)

AUTHOR

Libbey, L.M., and Sturtz, G.

TITLE

Unusual Essential Oils Grown in Oregon I. Artemisia afra Jacq.

PUBLICATION

J. Essent. Oil Res., Vol. 1, no. 1, 29-31 (1989)

COMPOUNDS

54.20%	-	alpha-Thujone	
13.70%	-	1, 8-Cineole	
13.70%	-	beta-Thujone	
8.80%	-	Camphor	
1.70%	-	Borneol	
1.60%	-	Camphene	
1.60%	-	Isoamyl isovalerate	
0.90%	-	Sesquiterpene hydrocarbons	
0.70%	-	Artemisia alcohol	
0.30%	-	Artemisia ketone	
0.10%	-	alpha-Pinene	
0.05%	-	para-Cymene	
97.35		TOTAL %	12 COMPOUNDS

Lanyana (South Africa)

BOTANICAL SPECIES

Artemisia afra Jacq., fam. Asteraceae (Compositae)

AUTHOR

Piprek, S.R.K., Graven, E.H., and Whitfield, P.

TITLE

Some Potentially Important Indigenous Aromatic Plants for the Eastern Seaboard areas of Southern Africa

PUBLICATION

in Aromatic Plants: Basic and Applied Aspects. H. Margaris, A. Koedam and D. Vokou, eds., Martinus Nijhoff Publ., The Hague, The Netheriands (1982)

COMPOUNDS

52.50%	-	alpha-Thujone	
13.10%	-	beta-Thujone	
13.00%	-	1, 8-Cineole	
6.55%	-	Camphor	
1.96%	-	Artemisia ketone	
1.62%	-	beta-Caryophyllene	
1.49%	-	alpha-Bergamotene	
1.38%	-	Aromadendrene	
1.15%	-	Camphene	
0.75%	-	gamma-Terpinene	
0.66%	-	para-Cymene	
0.51%	-	Terpinolene	
0.30%	-	alpha-Pinene	
94.97		TOTAL %	13 COMPOUNDS

Lanyana (Zimbabwe)

BOTANICAL SPECIES

Artemisia afra Jacq., fam. Asteraceae (Compositae)

AUTHOR

Moody, J.O., et al.

TITLE

Analysis of the Essential Oil of Artemisia afra

PUBLICATION

Pharmazie, Vol. 49, 935-936 (1994)

COMPOUNDS

19.03%	-	(Z)-2, 7-Dimethyl-4-octen-2, 7-diol
17.55%	-	1, 8-Cineole
13.92%	-	Tricosane
11.67%	-	3, 3, 6-Trimethyl-1, 5-heptadien-4-one
6.21%	-	Camphor
4.96%	-	Linalyl propionate
4.03%	-	alpha.p-Dimethylstyrene
2.67%	-	Isobomeol
1.66%	-	alpha-Thujone
1.22%	-	Terpinen-4-ol
1.19%	-	trans-Sabinene hydrate
0.99%	-	para-Cymene
0.91%	-	Camphene
0.84%	-	gamma-Elemene
0.73%	-	3-(Acetylmethyl)-beta-pinene
0.69%	-	alpha-Pinene
0.67%	-	beta-Santalol
0.55%	-	alpha-Thujene
89.49	TOTAL %	18 COMPOUNDS

Artemisia afra Willd. (Kenia)

BOTANICAL SPECIES

Artemisia afra Willd., fam. Asteraceae (Compositae)

AUTHOR

Mwangi, J.W., et al.

TITLE

Essential Oil Constituents of Artemisia afra Willd. (0.01 % = trace)

PUBLICATION

J. Essent. Oil Res., Vol. 7, 97-99 (1995)

COMPOUNDS

67.37%	-	1, 8-Cineole
6.50%	-	Terpinen-4-oi
5.09%	-	Borneol
2.30%	-	para-Cymene
2.00%	-	Isoamyl 2-methylbutyrate
1.64%	-	gamma-Terpinene
1.14%	-	l-Octenol-3
1.07%	-	trans-Verbenol
0.94%	-	alpha-Terpinyl acetate
0.76%	-	trans-p-Menth-2-en-1-ol
0.63%	-	cis-Sabinene hydrate
0.62%	-	alpha-Terpinene
0.58%	-	Caryophyllene oxide
0.43%	-	trans-Sabinene hydrate
0.32%	-	trans-Piperitol
0.27%	-	Limonene
0.24%	-	Isoamyl phenylacetate
0.23%	-	Bornyl acetate
0.18%	-	cis-p-Menth-2-en-l-ol

0.16%	-	beta-Pinene
0.12%	-	Camphene
0.09%	-	Sabinerie
0.09%	-	Spathulenol
0.06%	-	dehydro-1, 8-Cineole
0.05%	-	Terpinolene
0.01%	-	alpha-Phellandrene
0.01%	-	(Z)-beta-Ocimene
0.01%	-	Linalool
0.01%	-	alpha-Terpineol
0.01%	-	p-Cymen-8-ol
0.01%	-	Myrtenal
0.01%	-	trans-Pinocarveol
0.01%	-	delta-Terpineol
0.01%	-	Isoamyl isovalerate
0.01%	-	Pinocarvone
0.01%	-	cis-Verbenol
0.01%	-	Myrtenol
0.01%	-	(E)-Nerolidol
0.01%	-	Germacrer
0.01%	-	alpha-Cadinol
0.01%	-	Cuminaldehyde
0.01%	-	trans-Linalool oxide (5) (furanoid)
0.01%	-	cis-Linalool oxide (5) (furanoid)
0.01%	-	Terpinen-4-yl acetate
0.01%	-	2-Phenylethyl butyrate
0.01%	-	alpha, p-Dimethylstyrene
0.01%	-	Isoamyl isobutyrate
0.01%	-	cis, p-1(7),8-Menthadienol-2
0.01%	-	trans, p-1(7), 8-Menthadienol-2
0.01%	-	7-alpha-Silphiperfol-5-ene
93.13	TOTAL %	50 COMPOUNDS

Artemisia aksaiensis (China)

BOTANICAL SPECIES

Artemisia aksaiensis Y.R. Ling, fam. Asteraceae (Compositae)

AUTHOR

Liangfeng Zhu, Li Yonghua, Li Baoling, Lu Biyao & Xia Nianhe

TITLE

Aromatic Plants and Essential Constituents p. 273

PUBLICATION

South China institute of Botany, Chinese Academy of Sciences, Hai Feng Publishing Co., Chinese National Node forAPINMAP, distributed by Peace Book Co. Ltd., Hong Kong (1993)

COMPOUNDS

19.29%	-	1, 8-Cineole
15.03%	-	Camphor
6.17%	-	Terpinen-4-ol
5.44%	-	alpha-Thujone
2.18%	-	3, 6, 6-Trimethyl-2-norpinanol
2.10%	-	beta-Cubebene
1.31%	-	Piperitone
1.31%	-	Artemisia ketone
1.20%	-	Coumarin
1.13%	-	Borneol
1.10%	-	gamma-Elemene
0.42%	-	Sabinol
0.41%	-	alpha-Terpineol
0.41%	-	Cumin alcohol

0.32%	-	2-Hexenal	
0.31%	-	Umbellulone	
0.25%	-	para-Cymene	
0.20%	-	alpha-Terpinyl acetate	
0.18%	-	alpha-Terpinene	
58.76		TOTAL %	19 COMPOUNDS

Artemisia alba (Belgium)

BOTANICAL SPECIES

Artemisia alba Turra, fam. Asteraceae (Compositae)

AUTHOR

Ronse, A.C., and De Footer, H.L.

TITLE

Essential Oil Production by Belgian Artemisia alba (Turra) before and after Micropropargation (oil from mother plant)

PUBLICATION

J. Ess. Oil Res., Vol. 2, 237-242 (Sept./Oct. 1990)

COMPOUNDS

34.60%	-	Isopinocamphone
21.10%	-	Camphor
5.70%	-	1, 8-Cineole
4.10%	-	Camphene
3.80%	-	Myrtenol
3.40%	-	beta-Pinene
3.40%	-	T-Cadinol
3.00%	-	Myrtenal
1.50%	-	Pinocamphone
0.70%	-	delta-Cadinene
0.60%	-	Alkanes
0.50%	-	Terpinen-4-ol
0.50%	-	allo-Aromadendrene
0.20%	-	Borneol
0.10%	-	Pinocarvone
0.01%	-	Sabinene
0.01%	-	para-Cymene

0.01%	-	Carvone	
0.01%	-	beta-Caryophyllene	
0.01%	-	trans-Pinocarveol	
0.01%	-	Elemol	
0.01%	-	Germacrene D	
0.01%	-	Calamenene	
0.01%	-	alpha-Elemene	
83.29		TOTAL %	24 COMPOUNDS

Artemisia alba (Italy)

BOTANICAL SPECIES

Artemisia alba Turra, fam. Asteraceae (Compositae)

AUTHOR

Mucciarelli, M., Caramiello, R., Maffei, M., and Chialva, F.

TITLE

Essential Oils from Some Artemisia Species Growing Spontaneously in North-West Italy (0.01% = trace)

PUBLICATION

Flavour, Fragr. J., Vol. 10, 25-32 (1995)

COMPOUNDS

39.30%	-	Camphor
13.50%	-	Cuminaldehyde
10.20%	-	Isoplnocamphone
4.40%	-	Camphene
4.10%	-	Bornyl acetate
3.80%	-	Myrtenal
2.00%	-	trans-Pinocarveol
1.70%	-	Spathulenol
1.60%	-	beta-Pinene
1.40%	-	gamma-Selinene
1.20%	-	Irans-Carveol
1.10%	-	Caryophyllene oxide
0.90%	-	alpha-Pinene
0.70%	-	Terpinen-4-ol
0.70%	-	trans-Verbenol
0.70%	-	Carvacrol
0.60%	-	beta-Caryophyllene

0.40%	-	para-Cymene
0.40%	-	1, 8-Cineole
0.40%	-	Carvone
0.30%	-	alpha-Copaene
0.30%	-	Myrtenol
0.30%	-	Artemisyl acetate
0.20%	-	alpha-Thujene
0.20%	-	alpha-Terpinene
0.20%	-	alpha-Terpineol
0.20%	-	Artemisia alcohol
0.20%	-	Pinocarvone
0.20%	-	Verbenone
0.10%	-	Sabinene
0.10%	-	Limonene
0.10%	-	gamma-Terpinene
0.10%	-	Linalool
0.10%	-	beta-Thujone
0.10%	-	Yomogi alcohol
0.10%	-	Sabinene hydrate
0.10%	-	Linalool oxides (cis/trans) (unknown isomers)
0.10%	-	beta-Damascenone
0.10%	-	Camphenilone
0.10%	-	cis-2-Thujenol-4
0.01%	-	Myrcene
0.01%	-	alpha-Phellandrene
0.01%	-	Terpinolene
0.01%	-	Borneol
0.01%	-	alpha-Thujone
0.01%	-	dehydro-1, 8-Cineole
0.01%	-	(E)-Nerolidol

0.01%	-	alpha-Cadinol
0.01%	-	alpha-Fenchene
0.01%	-	alpha-Bisabolol
0.01%	-	Artemisia ketone
0.01%	-	cis-Chrysanthenyl acetate
0.01%	-	Ascaridole
0.01%	-	1-epi-Cubenol
0.01%	-	trans-alpha-Bergamotol
0.01%	-	Sabinyl acetate
0.01%	-	trans-Chrysantenyl acetate
0.01%	-	cis-Ocimene epoxide
0.01%	-	Nojigiku alcohol
0.01%	-	Bisabolol oxide (unknown isomer)
92.50		TOTAL % 60 COMPOUNDS

Artemisia anethifolia (China)

BOTANICAL SPECIES

Artemisia anethifolia Web. ex Stechm., fam. Asteraceae (Compositae)

AUTHOR

Liangfeng Zhu, Li Yonghua, Li Baoling, Lu Biyao & Xia Nianhe

TITLE

Aromatic Plants and Essential Constituents p. 274

PUBLICATION

South China Institute of Botany, Chinese Academy of Sciences, Hai Feng Publishing Co., Chinese National Node for APINMAP, distributed by Peace Book Co. Ltd., Hong Kong (1993)

COMPOUNDS

43.51%	-	1, 8-Cineole	
15.80%	-	Sabinol	
5.44%	-	Terpinen-4-ol	
3.66%	-	Borneol	
1.91%	-	Myrtenol	
1.30%	-	iso-Sabinol	
0.67%	-	beta-Selinene	
0.59%	-	p-lsopropylphenol	
0.49%	-	7-Octen-4-ol	
0.42%	-	gamma-Terpinene	
0.31%		para-Cymene	
0.20%	-	beta-Caryophyllene	
74.30		TOTAL %	12 COMPOUNDS

Artemisia anethoides (China)

BOTANICAL SPECIES

Artemisia anethoides Mattf., fam. Asteraceae (Compositae)

AUTHOR

Liangfeng Zhu, Li Yonghua, Li Baoling, Lu Biyao & Xia Nianhe

TITLE

Aromatic Plants and Essential Constituents p. 275

PUBLICATION

South China Institute of Botany, Chinese Academy of Sciences, Hai Feng Publishing Co., Chinese National Node for APINMAP, distributed by Peace Book Co. Ltd., Hong Kong (1993)

COMPOUNDS

64.27%	-	Piperitone
6.26%	-	1, 8-Cineole
3.59%	-	Davanone
1.04%	-	Artemisia ketone
0.88%	-	Terpinen-4-ol
0.86%	-	6-Methyl-3, 5-heptadien-2-one
0.74%	-	Cumin aicohol
0.73%	-	Linalool
0.68%	-	Camphor
0.64%	-	alpha-Terpineol
0.61%	-	Borneol
0.58%	-	5, 5-Dimethyl-2(5H)-furanone
0.10%	-	2-Hexenal
80.98	TOTAL %	13 COMPOUNDS

Annual wormwood (USA, Oregon)

BOTANICAL SPECIES

Artemisia annua L, fam. Asteraceae (Compositae)

AUTHOR

Libbey-, L.M., and Sturtz, G.

TITLE

Unusual Essential Oils Grown in Oregon II. Artemisia annua L.

PUBLICATION

J. Ess. Oil Res., Vol. 1, 201-202 (Sept./Oct., 1989)

COMPOUNDS

35.70%	-	Artemisia ketone
31.50%	-	1, 8-Cineole
11.20%	-	alpha-Pinene
5.20%	-	Artemisia alcohol
4.60%	-	Myrcene
2.50%	-	Sabinene
1.80%	-	beta-Pinene
1.30%	-	Pinocarvone
1.10%	-	trans-Pinocarveol
0.70%	-	Germacrene D
95.60		TOTAL % 10 COMPOUNDS

Annual wormwood (India)

BOTANICAL SPECIES

Artemisia annua L, fam. Asteraceae (Compositae)

AUTHOR

Thakur, R.S., and Misra, L.N.

TITLE

Essential Oils of Indian Artemisia

PUBLICATION

in: Proceedings 11th Intern. Congress of Essential Oils, Fragrances and Flavours, 12-16 Nov., 1989, New-Delhi, India, Vol. 4, 127-135

COMPOUNDS

38.40%	-	Borneol
14.40%	-	alpha-Terpineol
9.50%	-	Isoborneol
5.70%	-	Linalool
5.10%	-	Artemisia ketone
3.30%	-	Camphor
1.70%	-	Fenchone
1.60%	-	Tricyclene
0.10%	-	alpha-Pinene
0.05%	-	beta-Pinene
0.05%	-	beta-Caryophyllene
0.05%	-	beta-Farnesene
0.05%	-	alpha-Myrcene hydroperoxide
0.05%	-	beta-Myrcene hydroperoxide
0.05%	-	iso-Artemisia ketone
80.10	TOTAL %	15 COMPOUNDS

Annual wormwood 2

BOTANICAL SPECIES

Artemisia annua L., fam. Asteraceae (Compositae)

AUTHOR

Georgiev, E.V.; Genov, N.S., Lazarova, R.D., and Gantchev, G.P.

TITLE

On the distillation of annual wormwood (Artemisia annua L.)

PUBLICATION

Rivista Ital., Vol.60, 302-306 (1978)

COMPOUNDS

18.00%	-	Artemisia ketone
14.15%	-	Borneol
10.65%	-	Camphor
8.00%	-	beta-Caryophyllene
6.00%	-	Artemisia alcohol
4.75%	-	1, 8-Cineole
3.75%	-	Methyl chavicol
3.45%	-	Myrcene
2.55%	-	beta-Pinene
2.25%	-	Camphene
2.20%	-	alpha-Pinene
1.20%	-	para-Cymene
76.95	TOTAL %	12 COMPOUNDS

Annual wormwood 1

BOTANICAL SPECIES

Artemisia annua L, fam. Asteraceae (Compositae)

AUTHOR

Toleva, P.D. et al.

TITLE

Investigation on the essential oil of Artemisia annua

PUBLICATION

Paper no. 117, VIth int. Congress of Ess. Oils, San Francisco (Sept.Oct. 1974)

COMPOUNDS

64.00%	-	Artemisia ketone	
10.00%	-	alpha-Pinene	
7.00%	-	1, 8-Cineole	
5.00%	-	Camphor	
4.00%	-	Camphene	
2.00%	-	beta-Pinene	
2.00%	-	Artemisia alcohol	
2.00%	-	Menthol	
1.60%	-	alpha-Ylangene	
0.60%	-	Monoterpene alcohols	
0.50%	-	para-Cymene	
0.50%	-	(E)-beta-Ocimene	
0.50%	-	Artemisyl Acetate	
99.70		TOTAL %	13 COMPOUNDS

Annual wormwood, leaf (U.S.A., Indiana) 1

BOTANICAL SPECIES

Artemisia annua L., fam. Asteraceae (Compositae)

AUTHOR

Charles, D.J., Cebert, E., and Simon, J.E.

TITLE

Characterization of the Essential Oil of Artemisia annua L. (Leaf oil 1988; Plants harvested prior to flowering)

PUBLICATION

J. Ess. Oil Res., Vol. 3, 33-39 (Jan/Feb. 1991)

COMPOUNDS

35.60%	-	Artemisia ketone
28.10%	-	1, 8-Cineole
5.00%	-	beta-Caryophyllene
4.43%	-	beta-Cubebene
3.80%	-	Sabinene
3.80%	-	beta-Farnesene
2.31%	-	Camphene hydrate
2.02%	-	allo-Aromadendrene
1.90%	-	Artemisia alcohol
1.84%	-	Terpinen-4-ol
1.75%	-	Caryophyllene oxide
1.10%	-	alpha-Copaene
0.90%	-	Benzyl isovalerate
0.80%	-	beta-Pinene
0.71%	-	6-Melhyl-3, 5-heptadien-2-one
0.50%	-	alpha-Pinene
0.40%	-	alpha-Terpinene

0.40%	-	gamma-Elemene
0.28%	-	cis-Sabinene hydrate
0.20%	-	Myrtenal
0.20%	-	Santolinatriene
0.18%	-	beta-Cadinene
0.15%	-	alpha-Longipinene
0.14%	-	Sabina ketone
0.12%	-	alpha-Terpineol
0.10%	-	alpha-Thujene
0.10%	-	Myrtenol
0.04%	-	Isoeugenol
0.04%	-	p-Ethylcumene
0.03%	-	alpha-Humulene
96.94		TOTAL % 30 COMPOUNDS

Annual wormwood, leaf (U.S.A., Indiana) 2

BOTANICAL SPECIES

Artemisia annua L., fam. Asteraceae (Compositae)

AUTHOR

Charles, D.J., Cebert, E., and Simon, J.E

TITLE

Characterization of the Essential Oil of Artemisia annua L (Leaf oil 1987 Plants harvested after full bloom)

PUBLICATION

J. Ess. Oil Res., Vol. 3, 33-39 (Jan/Feb. 1991)

COMPOUNDS

26.85%	-	Artemisia ketone
20.48%	-	Camphor
8.70%	-	1, 8-Cineole
8.45%	-	allo-Aromadendrene
5.60%	-	beta-Caryophyllene
1.80%	-	beta-Cubebene
1.70%	-	Sabinol
1.55%	-	alpha-Copaene
1.40%	-	beta-Pinene
1.10%	-	Sabinene
0.95%	-	Caryophyllene oxide
0.94%	-	6-Methyl-3, 5-heptadien-2-one
0.84%	-	beta-Farnesene
0.72%	-	Artemisia alcohol
0.71%	-	alpha-Humulene
0.66%	-	gamma-Elemene
0.55%	-	Sabina ketone

0.50%	-	beta-Cadinene
0.50%	-	Myrtenal
0.40%	-	alpha-Pinene
0.36%	-	Benzyl isovalerate
0.33%	-	cis-Sabinene hydrate
0.33%	-	p-Ethylcumene
0.22%	-	alpha-Terpinene
0.15%	-	alpha-Longipinene
0.14%	-	Terpinen-4-ol
0.14%	-	Camphene hydrate
0.11%	-	Isoeugenol
0.10%	-	Myrtenol
0.08%	-	alpha-Terpineol
0.04%	-	Santolinatriene
0.01%	-	alpha-Thujene
86.41	TOTAL %	32 COMOUNDS

Annual wormwood, flower (U.S.A., Indiana)

BOTANICAL SPECIES

Artemisia annua L., fam. Asteraceae (Compositae)

AUTHOR

Charles, D.J., Cebert, E., and Simon, J.E.

TITLE

Characterization of the Essential Oil of Artemisia annua L. (Flower oil 1987)

PUBLICATION

J. Ess. Oil Res., Vol. 3, 33-39 (Jan/Feb. 1991)

COMPOUNDS

56.00%	-	Artemisia ketone
10.50%	-	Camphor
7.70%	-	1, 8-Cineole
3.30%	-	beta-Caryophyllene
3.26%	-	Caryophyllene oxide
2.60%	-	Sabinene
2.60%	-	beta-Farnesene
2.10%	-	Artemisia alcohol
2.09%	-	Camphene hydrate
1.20%	-	beta-Pinene
1.10%	-	Terpinen-4-ol
0.94%	-	beta-Cubebene
0.72%	-	Sabinol
0.61%	-	Benzyl isovaterate
0.40%	-	Myrtenal
0.37%	-	beta-Cadinene
0.31%	-	alpha-Copaene

0.24%	-	alpha-Pinene	
0.23%	-	Sabina ketone	
0.16%	-	Santolinatriene	
0.14%	-	Myrtenol	
0.13%	-	alpha-Thujene	
0.11%	-	gamma-Elemene	
0.10%	-	alpha-Longipinene	
0.09%	-	alpha-Terpineol	
0.06%	-	allo-Aromadendrene	
0.03%	-	Isoeugenol	
0.02%	-	p-Etnylcumene	
0.01%	-	alpha-Humulene	
97.12		TOTAL %	29 COMPOUNDS

Annual wormwood (Mongolia)

BOTANICAL SPECIES

Artemisia annua L, fam. Asteraceae (Compositae)

AUTHOR

Satar, S.

TITLE

Chemical characterization of essential oils from Mongolian species of the genus Artemisia L. (0.1% = estimated)

PUBLICATION

Pharmazie, Vol. 41, 819-820 (1986)

COMPOUNDS

40.00%	-	Thymol
40.00%	-	Carvacrol
4.40%	-	alpha-Terpineol
2.20%	-	Linalool
2.20%	-	Camphor
2.00%	-	Borneol
1.80%	-	1, 8-Cineote
1.70%	-	para-Cymene
0.70%	-	Limonene
0.50%	-	gamma-Terpinene
0.20%	-	delta-3-Carene
0.10%	-	alpha-Pinene
0.10%	-	Camphene
0.10%	-	Sabinene
0.16%	-	beta-Pinene
0.10%	-	Myrcene
0.10%	-	alpha-Terpinene
96.30	TOTAL %	17 COMPOUNDS

Annual wormwood (China) 1

BOTANICAL SPECIES

Artemisia annua L., fam. Asteraceae (Compositae)

AUTHOR

Liu, Q., Yang, Z., Sa, G., and Wang, X.

TITLE

Preliminary analysis of chemical constituents of essential oil from inflorenscence of Artemisia annua L.

PUBLICATION

Zhiwu Xuebao, Vol. 30, 223-225 (1988)

COMPOUNDS

63.10%	-	Artemisia ketone
1.92%	-	beta-Caryophyllene
1.50%	-	beta-Pinene
1.50%	-	1, 8-Cineole
0.90%	-	(E)-beta-Farnesene
0.70%	-	alpha-Copaene
0.70%	-	Benzyl isovalerate
0.40%	-	alpha-Longipinene
0.37%	-	beta-Phellandrene
0.36%	-	2-Methyl-6-methylene-1,7-octadien-3-one
0.31%	-	(E)-beta-Ocimene
0.30%	-	Nootkatone
0.30%	-	Cedrenol
0.20%	-	beta-Cadinene
0.20%	-	Jasmone
0.20%	-	1, 2, 3, 6-Tetramethylbicyclo[2.2.2]octa-2, 5-diene

0.18%	-	3-Methyl-3-butenyl 3-metnylbutyrate
0.16%	-	Terpinen-4-ol
0.12%	-	Hexane
0.11%	-	aipha-Terpineol
0.11%	-	Geraniol
0.10%	-	(Z)-3-Hexenyl propionate
0.06%	-	(E)-4-Methyl-2-hexene
0.05%	-	Ethyl 2-methylbutyrate
0.05%	-	Alloocimene (unknown isomer)
0.04%	-	alpha-Pinene
0.03%	-	(Z)-3-Hexenol
0.03%	-	Methylcyclopentane
0.02%	-	1-Hexanol
0.02%	-	3, 3-Dimethyl-1-butene
0.01%	-	Methyl 2-methylbutyrate
0.01%	-	3-Methylpentanal
0.01%	-	Heylcyclohexane
74.07	TOTAL %	33 COMPOUNDS

Annual wormwood (Yugoslavia)

BOTANICAL SPECIES

Artemisia annua L., fam. Asteraceae (Compositae)

AUTHOR

Chalchat, J.C., Garry, R.Ph., Michet, A., and Gorunovic, M.

TITLE

Essential oils of Artemisia annua from Yugoslavia (average of 2 oils)

PUBLICATION

Rivista Italiana EPPOS (Special Issue), 471-476 (1991)

COMPOUNDS

44.80%	-	Artemisia ketone
9.60%	-	1, 8-Cineole
6.30%	-	Camphor
6.20%	-	alpha-Ylangene
4.13%	-	alpha-Pinene
2.60%	-	Verbenone
2.00%	-	Camphene
1.90%	-	trans-Pinocarveol
1.88%	-	Artemisia alcohol
1.00%	-	Caryophyllene oxide
0.58%	-	para-Cymene
0.58%	-	Pinocarvone
0.58%	-	Menthol
0.38%	-	Methyl chamazulene
0.35%	-	Piperitol
0.33%	-	Carvone
0.30%	-	Cuminaldehyde
0.30%	-	Benzyl isovalerate

0.28%	-	trans-Verbenol
0.28%	-	Menthone
0.27%	-	Pinocamphone
0.25%	-	trans-Sabinene hydrate
0.25%	-	Ethyl 2-methylbutyrate
0.23%	-	Arteannuin B
0.20%	-	Borneol
0.20%	-	Bornyl acetate
0.15%	-	beta-Pinene
0.15%	-	p-Cymen-8-ol
0.15%	-	Artemisyl acetate
0.15%	-	Butyl 3-methylbutyrate
0.10%	-	Tricyclene
0.10%	-	T-Cadinol
0.10%	-	trans-Carveol
0.07%	-	alpha-Terpinene
0.05%"	-	Isopinocamphone
0.05%	-	2-Methyl-2-pentanol
0.05%	-	(E)-3, 3-Dimethylcyclohexylideneacetaldehyde
0.03%	-	Santolinatriene
0.03%	-	Acetone
0.01%	-	beta-Phellandrene
0.01%	-	l-Penten-4-ol
0.01%	-	Umbellulol
86.98	TOTAL %	42 COMPOUNDS

Annual wormwood (France)

BOTANICAL SPECIES

Artemisia annua L., fam. Asteraceae (Compositae)

AUTHOR

Chalchat, J.-C., R.-P. Garry & J. Lamy

TITLE

Influence of Harvest Time on Yield and Composition of Artemisia annua Oil Produced in France (oil sample no. 10, full flowering sep 20, 1990)

PUBLICATION

J. Essent. Oil Res, Vol. 6, 261-268 (1994)

COMPOUNDS

51.31%	-	Artemisia ketone
11.79%	-	1, 8-Cineole
5.05%	-	alpha-Pinene
4.94%	-	Camphor
3.24%	-	Myrcene
3.18%	-	Germacrene D
2.96%	-	alpha-Guaiene
2.63%	-	Sabinene
2.05%	-	beta-Cubebene
1.81%	-	Camphene
1.64%	-	beta-Caryophyllene
1.29%	-	beta-Pinene
0.91%	-	trans-Pinocarveol
0.88%	-	alpha-Thujene
0.43%	-	Yomogi alcohol
0.39%	-	cis-Sabinene hydrate

0.36%	-	Caryophyllene oxide
0.36%	-	Isocaryophyllene oxide
0.34%	-	trans-Sabinene hydrate
0.24%	-	Pinocarvone
0.23%	-	Bicyclogermacrene
0.19%	-	Terpinen-4-ol
0.18%	-	alpna-Terpinene
0.17%	-	Ethyl 2-methylbutyrate
0.15%	-	gamma-Terpinene
0.12%	-	Carvacrol
0.11%	-	Limonene
0.11%	-	(E)-beta-Ocimene
0.11%	-	delta-Cadinene
0.10%	-	alpha-Himachalene
0.09%	-	Tricyclene
0.09%	-	Santolina alcohol
0.08%	-	Thymol
0.06%	-	(E)-3, 3-Dimethylcyclohexylideneacetaldehyde
0.05%	-	Butyl 3-methylbutyrate
0.04%	-	para-Cymene
0.03%	-	alpha-Campholene aldehyde
0.03%	-	3-Methyl-3-butenyl 3-methylbutyrate
0.01%	-	Borneol
0.01%	-	Bornylene
0.01%	-	Myrtenal
0.01%	-	Spathulenol
0.01%	-	Cedrol
0.01%	-	Nootkatone
97.80	TOTAL %	44 COMPOUNDS

Annual wormwood (China) 2a

BOTANICAL SPECIES

Artemisia annua L, fam. Asteraceae (Compositae)

AUTHOR

Woerdenbag H.J., et al.

TITLE

Volatile constituents of Artemisia annua L. (Asteraceae) (analysis of steamdistilled oil)

PUBLICATION

Flav. Fragr. J., Vol. 8, 131-137 (1993)

COMPOUNDS

63.90%	-	Artemisia ketone
7.50%	-	Artemisia alcohol
5.10%	-	Myrcene
4.70%	-	alpha-Guaiene
3.30%	-	Camphor
2.50%	-	beta-Caryophyllene
1.30%	-	(E)-beta-Farnesene
0.90%	-	Yomogi alcohol
0.50%	-	cis-Sabinene hydrate
0.40%	-	alpha-Pinene
0.40%	-	Camphene
0.30%	-	cis-Chrysanthenol
0.30%	-	(E)-2, 7-Dimethylocta-4,6-dien-2-ol
0.20%	-	Borneol
0.10%	-	Isopinocamphone
0.10%	-	Artemisiatriene
0.05%	-	alpha-Thujene

0.05%	-	Sabinene	
0.05%	-	1, 8-Cineole	
0.05%	-	alpha-Humulene	
0.05%	-	Arteannuic acid	
0.01%	-	beta-Pinene	
91.76		TOTAL %	22 COMPOUNDS

Annual wormwood (China) 2b

BOTANICAL SPECIES

Artemisia annua L., fam. Asteraceae (Compositae)

AUTHOR

Woerdenbag H.J., et al.

TITLE

Volatile constituents of Artemisia annua L. (Asteraceae) (analysis of methyiene chloride extract)

PUBLICATION

Flav. Fragr. J., Vol. 8, 131-137 (1993)

COMPOUNDS

49.90%	-	Artemisia ketone
5.30%	-	Artemisia alcohol
4.90%	-	Camphor
3.50%	-	Arteannuic acid
3.30%	-	alpha-Guaiene
3.20%	-	Arteannuin B
2.10%	-	Myrcene
1.70%	-	Artemisinin
1.60%	-	beta-Myrcene hydroperoxide
1.50%	-	alpha-Myrcene hydroperoxide
1.00%	-	Camphene
0.50%	-	beta-Caryophyllene
0.40%	-	alpha-Pinene
0.40%	-	Yomogi alcohol
0.30%	-	(E)-beta-Farnesene
0.20%	-	beta-Pinene
0.20%	-	Borneol

0.20%	-	cis-Sabinene hydrate	
0.20%	-	cis-Chrysanthenol	
0.20%	-	(E)-2, 7-Dimethylocta-4,6-dien-2-ol	
0.10%	-	Artemisiatriene	
0.05%	-	alpha-Thujene	
0.05%	-	Sabinene	
0.05%	-	Isopinocamphone	
80.85		TOTAL %	24 COMPOUNDS

Annual wormwood (Vietnam) 1a

BOTANICAL SPECIES

Artemisia annua L., fam. Asteraceae (Compositae)

AUTHOR

Woerdenberg, H.J., et al.

TITLE

Volatile constituents of Artemisia annua L. (analysis of steamdistilled oil)

PUBLICATION

Flav. Fragr. J., Vol. 8, 131-137 (1993)

COMPOUNDS

21.80%	-	Camphor
16.30%	-	Germacrene D
5.60%	-	beta-Caryophyllene
3.80%	-	(E)-beta-Farnesene
3.10%	-	1, 8-Cineole
2.30%	-	Camphene
1.70%	-	Cadinol (unknown structure)
1.50%	-	gamma-Elemene
1.30%	-	Borneol
0.70%	-	para-Cymene
0.70%	-	alpha-Copaene
0.60%	-	alpha-Guaiene
0.50%	-	alpha-Pinene
0.50%	-	Terpinen-4-ol
0.50%	-	cis-Chrysanthenol
0.40%	-	Neryl acetate
0.30%	-	alpha-Humulene

0.30%	-	cis-Chrysanthenyl acetate
0.30%	-	trans-Chrysantenyl acetate
0.20%	-	beta-Elemene
0.10%	-	beta-Pinene
0.10%	-	alpha-Terpineol
0.10%	-	Bornyl acetate
0.05%	-	alpha-Thujene
0.05%	-	Sabinene
0.05%	-	gamma-Terpinene
0.05%	-	trans-Sabinene hydrate
0.05%	-	cis-Sabinene hydrate
0.05%	-	Arteannuic acid
65.00	TOTAL %	29 COMPOUNDS

Annual wormwood (Hungary)

BOTANICAL SPECIES

Artemisia annua L., fam. Asteraceae (Compositae)

AUTHOR

Hethelyi, E.B., et al.

TITLE

Chemical composition of the Artemisia anua Essential Oils from Hungry (average analysis of 35 samples)

PUBLICATION

J. Essent. Oil Res., Vol. 7, 45-8 (Jan/Feb 1995)

COMPOUNDS

64.00%	-	Artemisia ketone
24.00%	-	Artemisia alcohol
3.00%	-	Yomogi alcohol
2.00%	-	beta-Pinene
2.00%	-	alpha-Cubebene
1.50%	-	para-Cymene
1.00%	-	alpha-Pinene
1.00%	-	1, 8-Cineole
1.00%	-	Camphor
99.50	TOTAL %	9 COMPOUNDS

Annual wormwood (Italy)

BOTANICAL SPECIES

Artemisia annua L, fam. Asteraceae (Compositae)

AUTHOR

Mucciarelli, M., Caramiello, R., Maffei, M., and Chialva, F.

TITLE

Essential Oils from Some Artemisia Species Growing Spontaneously in North-West Italy (0.01% = trace)

PUBLICATION

Flavour Fragr. J, Vol. 10, 25-32 (1995)

COMPOUNDS

23.30%	-	1, 8-Cineole
19.60%	-	alpha-Pinene
15.50%	-	Camphor
7.30%	-	Caryophyllene oxide
5.50%	-	Pinocarveol
4.10%	-	Carvacrol
3.50%	-	gamma-Selinene
2.40%	-	Camphene
2.10%	-	beta-Pinene
2.00%	-	Terpinen-4-ol
1.80%	-	alpha-Terpineol
1.40%	-	Myrcene
1.10%	-	Sabinene
1.00%	-	para-Cymene
1.00%	-	Borneol
1.00%	-	Ascaridole
0.70%	-	gamma-Terpinene

0.70%	-	beta-Caryophyllene
0.60%	-	Myrtenol
0.60%	-	Verbenone
0.50%	-	Myrtenal
0.50%	-	trans-Verbenol
0.50%	-	Bisabolol oxide (unknown isomer)
0.40%	-	alpha-Terpinene
0.40%	-	Cuminaldehyde
0.30%	-	Carvone
0.30%	-	alpha-Copaene
0.30%	-	Linalool oxides (cis/trans) (unknown isomers)
0.30%	-	cis-2-Thujenol-4
0.20%	-	Limonene
0.20%	-	Terpinolene
0.20%	-	Pinocarvone
0.20%	-	Sabinene hydrate
0.20%	-	(E)-Nerolidol
0.10%	-	dehydro-1, 8-Cineole
0.10%	-	beta-Damascenone
0.10%	-	Nojigiku alcohol
0.01%	-	alpha-Thujene
0.01%	-	alpha-Phellandrene
0.01%	-	Linalool
0.01%	-	Bornyl acetate
0.01%	-	alpha-Thujone
0.01%	-	beta-Thujone
0.01%	-	Yomogi alcohol
0.01%	-	Artemisia alcohol
0.01%	-	Spathulenol
0.01%	-	alpha-Cadinol

0.01%	-	alpha-Fenchene
0.01%	-	trans-Carveol
0.01%	-	alpha-Bisabolol
0.01%	-	Artemisia ketone
0.01%	-	Artemisyl acetate
0.01%	-	cis-Chrysanthenyl acetate
0.01%	-	1-epi-Cubenol
0.01%	-	Camphenilone
0.01%	-	Isopinocamphone
0.01%	-	trans-alpha-Bergamotol
0.01%	-	Sabinyl acetate
0.01%	-	trans-Chrysantenyl acetate
0.01%	-	cis-Ocimene epoxide
100.23	TOTAL %	60 COMPOUNDS

Artemisia arborescens (U.S.A.)

BOTANICAL SPECIES

Artemisia arborescens L, fam. Asteraceae (Compositae)

AUTHOR

Tucker, A.O., M.J. Maciarello & G. Sturtz

TITLE

The Essential Oils of Artemisia 'Powis Castle' and its Putative Parents, A. absinthium and A. arborescens (analysis of field-distilled oil)

PUBLICATION

J. Essent. Oil Res., Vol.5, 239-242 (May/Jun 1993)

COMPOUNDS

21.39%	-	Chamazulene
17.39%	-	Camphor
6.43%	-	Terpinen-4-ol
6.38%	-	gamma-Terpinene
6.11%	-	Germacrene D
5.82%	-	alpha-Pinene
4.61%	-	Camphene
3.98%	-	alpha-Terpinene
2.73%	-	trans-Sabinene hydrate
2.69%	-	Limonene
1.73%	-	Terpinolene
0.72%	-	Sabinene
0.65%	-	alpha-Copaene
0.54%	-	para-Cymene
0.43%	-	Caryophyllene oxide
0.42%	-	alpha-Phellandrene

0.41%	-	1, 8-Cineole	
0.36%	-	beta-Pinene	
0.17%	-	beta-Thujone	
0.15%	-	6-Methyl-5-hepten-2-one	
0.06%	-	alpha-Thujone	
83.17		TOTAL %	21 COMPOUNDS

Artemisia argentea (Madeira)

BOTANICAL SPECIES

Artemisia argentea L'Her., fam. Asteraceae (Compositae)

AUTHOR

Fiqueiredo,A.C.,J.G.Barroso,L.G.Pedro,S.S. Fontinha,A. Looman & J.Scheffer

TITLE

Composition of the Essential Oil of Artemisia argentea L'Her., an Endemic Species of the Madeira Archipelago (analysis of leaf oil)

PUBLICATION

Flavour Fragr. J., Vol. 9, 229-232 (1994)

COMPOUNDS

27.30%	-	alpha-Phellandrene
8.10%	-	beta-Caryophyllene
7.60%	-	beta-Eudesmol
7.00%	-	Isopinocamphone
6.40%	-	beta-Pinene
6.30%	-	para-Cymene
4.70%	-	Pinocarvone
3.60%	-	Myrcene
3.20%	-	Germacrene D
2.80%	-	Geranyl 3-methylbutyrate
2.10%	-	1, 8-Cineoie
1.70%	-	Caryophyllene oxide
1.30%	-	trans-Pinocarveol
1.30%	-	Geranyl 2-methylbutyrate
1.10%	-	Sabinene
1.00%	-	Linalool

0.90%	-	alpha-Humulene
0.90%	-	Spathulenol
0.90%	-	Humulene oxide
0.80%	-	alpha-Pinene
0.80%	-	Limonene
0.70%	-	beta-Selinene
0.70%	-	gamma-Cadinene
0.70%	-	Bicyclogermacrene
0.60%	-	alpha-Copaene
0.50%	-	Myrtenol
0.50%	-	beta-Bourbonene
0.40%	-	(E)-2-Hexenal
0.30%	-	alpha-Cadinol
0.20%	-	(E)-beta-Ocimene
0.20%	-	alpha-Terpineol
0.20%	-	delta-Cadinene
0.20%	-	Phenylacetaldehyde
0.01%	-	alpha-Thujene
0.01%	-	alpha-Terpinene
0.01%	-	gamma-Terpinene
0.01%	-	Terpinen-4-ol
0.01%	-	alpha-Muurolene
0.01%	-	beta-Thujone
0.01%	-	trans-Sabinene hydrate
0.01%	-	beta-Elemene
0.01%	-	alpha-Farnesene
0.01%	-	trans-Carveol
0.01%	-	Cuminaldehyde
0.01%	-	Chamazulene
0.01%	-	Campholenal
95.13	TOTAL %	46 COMPOUNDS

Arternisia atrovirens (China)

BOTANICAL SPECIES

Arternisia atrovirens Hand.-Mazz., fam. Asteraceae (Compositae)

AUTHOR

Liangfeng Zhu, Li Yonghua, Li Baoling, Lu Biyao & Xia Nianhe

TITLE

Aromatic Plants and Essential Constituents p. 276

PUBLICATION

South China institute of Botany, Chinese Academy of Sciences, Hai Feng Publishing Co., Chinese National Node for APINMAP, distributed by Peace Book Co. Ltd., Hong Kong (1993)

COMPOUNDS

20.97%	-	Arternisia ketone
10.51%	-	1, 8-Cineole
4.33%	-	alpha-Bisabolol oxide B
2.75%	-	Camphor
2.43%	-	beta-Caryophyllene
1.76%	-	7-Octen-4-ol
1.72%	-	beta-Farnesene
1.52%	-	Naphthalene
1.51%	-	beta-Cubebene
1.15%	-	Borneol
1.14%	-	Linalool
1.14%	-	3-Hexenyl butyrate
1.10%	-	3, 6, 6-Trimethyl-2-norpinanol
1.06%	-	Nerolidol (unknown isomer)
0.99%	-	alpha-Humulene

0.98%	-	alpha-Bisabolol	
0.93%	-	Myrtenol	
0.77%	-	Eremophilene	
0.67%	-	Hexanal	
0.57%	-	Terpinen-4-ol	
0.56%	-	2-Hexenal	
0.45%	-	alpha-Terpineol	
59.01		TOTAL %	22 COMPOUNDS

Artesimia campestris (Italy) 2

BOTANICAL SPECIES

Artemisia campestris L. ssp campestris, fam. Asteraceae (Compositae)

AUTHOR

Mucciarelii, M., Caramieilo, R., Maffei, M., and Chialva, F.

TITLE

Essential Oils from Some Artemisia Species Growing Spontaneously in North-West Italy (0.01% = trace)

PUBLICATION

Flavour Fragr. J., Vol. 10, 25-32 (1995)

COMPOUNDS

19.20%	-	1, 8-Cineole
18.70%	-	Spathulenol
16.50%	-	alpha-Pinene
14.10%	-	1-epi-Cubenol
10.70%	-	beta-Pinene
5.70%	-	Caryophyllene oxide
5.30%	-	Sesquiterpene alcohols (unknown)
4.70%	-	Cuminaldehyde
2.70%	-	Camphor
2.70%	-	Pinocarveol
2.40%	-	Verbenone
2.20%	-	trans-alpha-Bergamotol
1.80%	-	isopinocamphone
1.70%	-	Limonene
1.50%	-	Carvacrol
1.30%	-	Borneol

1.10%	-	trans-Verbenol
0.90%	-	para-Cymene
0.90%	-	beta-Thujone
0.90%	-	Myrtenal
0.90%	-	Pinocarvone
0.60%	-	Camphene
0.40%	-	Sabinene
0.30%	-	Myrcene
0.30%	-	alpha-Terpineol
0.30%	-	dehydro-1, 8-Cineole
0.01%	-	alpha-Thujene
0.01%	-	alpha-Phellandrene
0.01%	-	alpha-Terpinene
0.01%	-	gamma-Terpinene
0.01%	-	Terpinolene
0.01%	-	Linalool
0.01%	-	Terpinen-4-ol
0.01%	-	Carvone
0.01%	-	Bornyl acetate
0.01%	-	beta-Caryophyllene
0.01%	-	beta-Selinene
0.01%	-	alpha-Copaene
0.01%	-	alpha-Thujone
0.01%	-	Yomogi alcohol
0.01%	-	Artemisia alcohol
0.01%	-	Myrtenol
0.01%	-	Sabinene hydrate
0.01%	-	(E)-Nerolidol
0.01%	-	alpha-Cadinol
0.01%	-	alpha-Fenchene
0.01%	-	trans-Carveol

0:01%	-	alpha-Bisabolol
0.01%	-	Artemisia ketone
0.01%	-	Artemisyl acetate
0.01%	-	cis-Chrysanthenyl acetate
0.01%	-	Linalool oxides (cis/trans) (unknown isomers)
0.01%	-	beta-Damascenone
0.01%	-	Ascaridole
0.01%	-	Camphenilone
0.01%	-	Sabinyl acetate
0.01%	-	trans-Chrysantenyl acetate
0.01%	-	cis-Ocimene epoxide
0.01%	-	cis-2-Thujenol-4
0.01%	-	Nojigiku alcohol
0.01%	-	Bssabolol oxide (unknown isomer)
118.15	TOTAL %	61 COMPOUNDS

Artemisia chamaemelifolia (Italy)

BOTANICAL SPECIES

Artemisia chamaemelifolia Vill., fam. Asteraceae (Compositae)

AUTHOR

Mucciarelli, M., Caramiello, R., Maffei, M., and Chialva, F.

TITLE

Essential Oils from Some Artemisia Species Growing Spontaneously in North-West Italy (0.01% = trace)

PUBLICATION

Flavour Fragr. J, Vol. 10, 25-32 (1995)

COMPOUNDS

22.60%	-	(E)-Nerolidol
22.60%	-	Sesquiterpene alcohols (unknown)
16.30%	-	Carvacrol
15.30%	-	1, 8-Cineole
3.40%	-	Spathulenol
3.00%	-	alpha-Bisabolol
3.00%	-	Bisabolol oxide (unknown isomer)
1.50%	-	alpha-Thujone
1.40%	-	Terpinen-4-ol
0.50%	-	alpha-Terpineol
0.50%	-	Caryophyllene oxide
0.40%	-	para-Cymene
0.40%	-	gamma-Terpinene
0.30%	-	Myrtenal
0.30%	-	Myrtenol
0.30%	-	Sabinene hydrate

0.30% - Cuminaldehyde
0.20% - Sabinene
0.20% - alpha-Terpinene
0.20% - Pinocarvone
0.20% - Sabinyl acetate
0.20% - cis-2-Thujenol-4
0.10% - alpha-Thujene
0.10% - Limonene
0.10% - Terpinolene
0.10% - Linalool
0.10% - Camphor
0.10% - beta-Caryophyllene
0.10% - alpha-Copaene
0.10% - beta-Thujone
0.10% - dehydro-1, 8-Cineole
0.10% - Pinocarveol
0.10% - gamma-Selinene
0.01% - alpha-Pinene
0.01% - Camphene
0.01% - beta-Pinene
0.01% - Myrcene
0.01% - alpha-Phellandrene
0.01% - Borneol
0.01% - Carvone
0.01% - Bornyl acetate
0.01% - Yomogi alcohol
0.01% - Artemisia alcohol
0.01% - trans-Verbenol
0.01% - alpha-Cadinol
0.01% - Verbenone
0.01% - alpha-Fenchene

0.01%	-	trans-Carveol	
0.01%	-	Artemisia ketone	
0.01%	-	Artemisyl acetate	
0.01%	-	cis-Chrysanthenyl acetate	
0.01%	-	Linalool oxides (cis/trans) (unknown isomers)	
0.01%	-	beta-Damascenone	
0.01%	-	Ascaridole	
0.01%	-	1-epi-Cubenol	
0.01%	-	Camphenilone	
0.01%	-	Isopinocamphone	
0.01%	-	trans-alpha-Bergamotol	
0.01%	-	trans-Chrysantenyl acetate	
0.01%	-	cis-Ocimene epoxide	
0.01%	-	Nojigiku alcohol	
94.48		TOTAL %	61 COMPOUNDS

Artemisia desertorum (China)

BOTANICAL SPECIES

Artemisia desertorum Spreng., fam. Aseraceae (Compositae)

AUTHOR

Liangfeng Zhu, Li Yonghua,Li Baoling, Lu Biyao & Xia Nianhe

TITLE

Aromatic plants and Essential Constituents p. 277

PUBLICATION

South China Institute of Botany, Chinese Academy of Sciences, Hai Feng Publishing Co., Chinese National Node for APINMAP, distributed by Peace book Co. Ltd., Hong Kong (1993)

COMPOUNDS

55.53%	-	alpha-Bisabolol	
14.00%	-	alpha-Bisabolol oxide B	
2.92%	-	Jasmone	
0.48%	-	Citronellyl acetate	
0.44%	-	Sabinol	
0.40%	-	m-Cresol	
0.39%	-	alpha-Curcumene	
0.33%	-	Citronellyl propionate	
74.49		TOTAL %	8 COMPOUNDS

Tarragon (USA) 1

BOTANICAL SPECIES

Artemisia dracunculus L., (French tarragon), fam. Asteraceae (Compositae)

AUTHOR

Tucker, A.O., and Madareiio, M.J.

TITLE

Plant Identification (oil from fresh leaves)

PUBLICATION

In: Proceedings of the First National Herb Growing and Marketing Conference, Edits. J.E. Simon and L. Grant, Purdue Univ. Press, West Lafayette IN (1987), pp 126-172

COMPOUNDS

80.02%	-	Methyl chavicol
7.00%	-	(E)-beta-Ocimene
6.59%	-	(Z)-beta-Ocimene
2 53%	-	Limonene
0.59%	-	alpha-Pinene
0.46%	-	Methyl eugenol
0.47%	-	gamma-Terpinene
0.26%	-	Eugenol
0.12%	-	Myrcene
0.12%	-	Methyl isoeugenol
0.09%	-	beta-Pinene
0.08%	-	Sabinene
0.06%	-	Linalool
0.05%	-	Elemicin
0.04%	-	Camphene
0.04%	-	Terpinolene
0.04%	-	Geraniol
0.03%	-	Nerol
0.03%	-	trans-Alloocimene

0.02%	-	Terpinen-4-ol
0.02%	-	1, 8-Cineole
0.02%	-	trans-Isoelemicin
0.01%	-	alpha-Thujene
0.01%	-	alpha-Pheiiandrene
0.01%	-	alpha-Terpinene
0.01%	-	para-Cymene
0.01%	-	Citronellyl acetate
0.00%	-	cis-Alloocimene
98.75	TOTAL %	28 COMPOUNDS

Tarragon (USA) 2

BOTANICAL SPECIES

Artemisia dracunculus L., (French tarragon), fam. Asteraceae (Compositae)

AUTHOR

Tucker, A.O., and Maciarello, M J.

TITLE

Plant Identification (oil from dried leaves)

PUBLICATION

In: Proceedings of the First National Herb Growing and Marketing Conference, Edits. J.E. Simon and L. Grant, Purdue Univ. Press, West Lafayette IN (1987), pp. 126-172

COMPOUNDS

59.77%	-	Methyl chavicol
10.00%	-	(E)-beta-Ocimene
9.33%	-	(Z)-beta-Ocimene
3.97%	-	Limonene
1.34%	-	alpha-Pinene
0.82%	-	Methyl eugenol
0.82%	-	Methyl isoeugenol
0.74%	-	Elemicin
0.55%	-	gamma-Terpinene
0.54%	-	Eugenol
0.21%	-	Nerol
0.20%	-	Myrcene
0.19%	-	Geraniol
0.14%	-	beta-Pinene
0.11%	-	Sabinene
0.06%	-	Linalool

0.05%	-	Terpinolene
0.04%	-	Camphene
0.04%	-	trans-Alloocimene
0.03%	-	Terpinen-4-ol
0.02%	-	1, 8-Cineole
0.02%	-	Citronellyl acetate
0.02%	-	trans-Isoelemicin
0.01%	-	alpha-Thujene
0.01%	-	alpha-Phellandrene
0.01%	-	alpha-Terpinene
0.01%	-	para-Cymene
0.01%	-	cis-Alloocimene
89.06	TOTAL %	28 COMPOUNDS

Tarragon (USA) 3

BOTANICAL SPECIES

Artemisia dracunculus L., (Russian type), fam. Asteraceae (Compositae)

AUTHOR

Tucker, A.O., and Maciarello, M.J.

TITLE

Plant identification (average concentrations of oils from fresh and dried leaves from clone 1)

PUBLICATION

In: Proceedings of the First National Herb Growing and Marketing Conference, Edits. J.E. Simon and L. Grant, Purdue Univ. Press, West Lafayette IN (1987), pp 126-172

COMPOUNDS

46.87%	-	Sabinene
17.48%	-	trans-Isoelemicin
8.27%	-	Methyl eugenol
4.23%	-	(Z)-beta-Ocimene
3.80%	-	(E)-beta-Ocimene
2.86%	-	Methyl isoeugenol
2.48%	-	Terpinen-4-ol
2.45%	-	Myrcene
1.25%	-	Citronellyl acetate
0.86%	-	alpha-Terpinene
0.55%	-	alpha-Pinene
0.53%	-	beta-Pinene
0.52%	-	Eiemicin
0.43%	-	Eugenol
0.33%	-	Terpinolene

0.21%	-	1, 8-Cineole	
0.19%	-	Camphene	
0.17%	-	Limonene	
0.10%	-	gamma-Terpinene	
0.10%	-	Linalool	
0.06%	-	Nerol	
0.06%	-	Methyl chavicol	
0.04%	-	Geraniol	
0.03%	-	alpha-Phellandrene	
0.03%	-	para-Cymene	
0.02%	-	trans-Alloocimene	
0.01%	-	alpha-Thujene	
0.01%	-	cis-Alloocimene	
93.94		TOTAL %	28 COMPOUNDS

Tarragon (USA) 4

BOTANICAL SPECIES

Artemisia dracunculus L., (Russian type), fam. Asteraceae (Compositae)

AUTHOR

Tucker, A.O., and Maciarello, M.J.

TITLE

Plant Identifications (average concentrations of oils from fresh and dried leaves from clone 2)

PUBLICATION

In: Proceedings of the First National Herb Growing and Marketing Conference, Edits. J.E. Simon and L. Grant, Purdue Univ. Press, West Lafayette IN (1987), pp 126-172

COMPOUNDS

52.23%	-	Elemicin
19.40%	-	Sabinene
7.77%	-	Methyl eugenol
5.00%	-	(E)-beta-Ocimene
1.90%	-	(Z)-beta-Ocimene
1.80%	-	Citronellyl acetate
1.47%	-	Terpinen-4-ol
1.41%	-	Terpinolene
0.87%	-	Myrcene
0.30%	-	gamma-Terpinene
0.27%	-	alpha-Terpinene
0.26%	-	trans-isoelemicin
0.21%	-	Methyl chavicol
0.13%	-	Limonene
0.12%	-	alpha-Pinene

0.11%	-	Lmalool
0.11%	-	1, 8-Cineole
0.10%	-	Eugenol
0.08%	-	beta-Pinene
0.07%	-	Camphene
0.06%	-	alpha-Phellandrene
0.06%	-	Nerol
0.05%	-	Methyl isoeugenol
0.04%	-	para-Cymene
0.03%	-	trans-Alloocimene
0.02%	-	alpha-Thujene
0.02%	-	cis-Alloocimene
93.89	TOTAL %	27 COMPOUNDS

Estragon

BOTANICAL SPECIES

Artemisia dracunculus L., fam. Asteraceae (Compositae)

AUTHOR

Vostrowsky, O., et al.

TITLE

Chemical Composition of Estragon oil

PUBLICATION

Z. Lebensmittel-Unters.u.-Forsch., Vol. 173, 365-367, (1981)

COMPOUNDS

38.81%	-	Sabinene
28.87%	-	Methyl eugenol
17.26%	-	Methyl chavicol
1.62%	-	Mycrene
1.15%	-	Methyl isoeugenol
0.89%	-	Citronellyl acetate
0.50%	-	alpha-Terpinene
0.45%	-	Geranyl acetate
0.34%	-	Elemicin
0.26%	-	Terpinolene
0.16%	-	alpha-Thujene
0.14%	-	Cinnamyl acetate
0.05%	-	Bornyl acetate
0.03%	-	alpha-Pinene
90.53	TOTAL %	14 COMPOUNDS

Tarragon (France) 1

BOTANICAL SPECIES

Artemisia dracunculus L., fam. Asteraceae (Compositae)

AUTHOR

Baritaux, O., et al.

PUBLICATION

Rivista Ital. EPPOS, (Numero speciale), 416-426 (1992)

COMPOUNDS

73.20%	-	Methyl chavicol
13.50%	-	(E)-beta-Ocimene
10.00%	-	(Z)-beta-Ocimene
1.80%	-	Limonene
0.70%	-	Methyl eugenol
0.40%	-	alpha-Pinene
0.30%	-	Eugenol
99.90		TOTAL % 7 COMPOUNDS

Tarragon (France) 2

BOTANICAL SPECIES

Artemisia dracunculus L., fam. Asteraceae (Compositae)

AUTHOR

Piccaglia, R., et al.

TITLE

Antibacterial and antioxidant properties of Mediterranean aromatic plants

PUBLICATION

Indust. Crops products, (20,47-50 (1993)

COMPOUNDS

77.50%	-	Methyl chavicol	
7.00%	-	(Z)-beta-Ocimene	
7.00%	-	(E)-beta-Ocimene	
1.50%	-	alpha-Pinene	
93.00		TOTAL %	4 COMPOUNDS

Tarragon (Italy)

BOTANICAL SPECIES

Artemisia dracunculus L., fam. Asteraceae (Compositae)

AUTHOR

Tateo, F., Santamaria, L., Bianchi, L. and Bianchi, A.

TITLE

Basil Oil and Tarragon Oil: Composition and Genotoxicity Evaluation

PUBLICATION

J. Ess. Oil Res, Vol. 1, 111-118, (May/June, 1989)

COMPOUNDS

60.46%	-	Methyl chavicol
17.01%	-	gamma-Terpinene
13.54%	-	(Z)-beta-Ocimene
4.65%	-	Limonene
1.44%	-	alpha-Pinene
0.64%	-	Sesquiterpene hydrocarbons (unknown)
0.51%	-	Methyl eugenol
0.30%	-	Eugenol
0.25%	-	Myrcene
0.19%	-	beta-Pinene
0.14%	-	Sabinene
0.14%	-	Cinnamyl acetate
0.14%	-	Menthone
0.11%	-	Camphene
0.11%	-	p-Methoxycinnamaldehyde
0.09%	-	alpha-Thujone
0.09%	-	beta-Thujone
0.03%	-	Linalool
0.01%	-	alpha-Thujene
99.85		TOTAL % 19 COMPOUNDS

Tarragon

BOTANICAL SPECIES

Artemisia dracunculus L, fam. Asteraceae (Compositae)

AUTHOR

Werker, E., et al.

TITLE

Glandular hairs, secretory cavities and essential oils in leaves of tarragon (Artemisia dracunculus L.) (analysis of hydrodist. oil of whole leaf)

PUBLICATION

J. Herbs, Spices Med. Plants, Vol 2 (3), 19-32 (1994)

COMPOUNDS

77.00%	-	Methyl chavicol
9.00%	-	(E)-bela-Ocimene
8.10%	-	(Z)-beta-Ocimene
2.50%	-	Limonene
0.90%	-	gamma-Terpinene
0.50%	-	Eugenol
0.50%	-	Methyl eugenol
0.20%	-	Nerol
0.20%	-	Elemicin
0.10%	-	beta-Pinene
0.10%	-	Myrcene
0.10%	-	para-Cymene
0.10%	-	Linalool
0.10%	-	Terpinen-4-ol
0.10%	-	Geraniol
0.05%	-	alpha-Pinene

0.05%	-	Camphene
0.05%	-	Sabinene
0.05%	-	alpna-Terpinene
0.05%	-	Terpinolene
0.05%	-	1, 8-Cineole
99.80	TOTAL %	21 COMPOUNDS

Tarragon (Cuba)

BOTANICAL SPECIES

Artemisia dracunculus L., fam. Asteraceae (Compositae)

AUTHOR

Pino, J.A., et al.

TITLE

Chemical Composition of the Essential Oil of Artemisia dracunculus L. from Cuba

PUBLICATION

J. Essent. Oil Res, Vol. 8, 563-564 (Sep/Oct 1996)

COMPOUNDS

53.03%	-	Elemicin
17.61%	-	Methyl eugenol
4.53%	-	Sabinene
3.95%	-	Terpinen-4-ol
2.60%	-	Isoelemicin
2.10%	-	Citronellol
2.00%	-	gamma-Terpinene
1.59%	-	alpha-Himachalene
0.94%	-	alpha-Thujene
0.88%	-	alpha-Terpinene
0.88%	-	para-Cymene
0.77%	-	beta-Phellandrene
0.73%	-	beta-Pinene
0.54%	-	Terpinolene
0.51%	-	beta-Caryophyllene
0.49%	-	Methyl chavicol
0.43%	-	trans-Sabinene hydrate
0.34%	-	cis-Sabinene hydrate

0.34%	-	(Z)-beta-Farnesene
0.30%	-	(Z)-beta-Ocimene
0.29%	-	alpha-Humulene
0.27%	-	(E, Z)-alpha-Farnesene
0.25%	-	(E)-beta-Ocimene
0.21%	-	alpha-Pinene
0.14%	-	Linalool
0.13%	-	alpha-Phellandrene
0.12%	-	alpha-Terpineol
0.11%	-	delta-Cadinene
0.10%	-	Menthone
0.08%	-	Carvacrol
0.08%	-	(E)-Cinnamic alcohol
0.07%	-	cis-Rose oxide
0.05%	-	Geranial
0.04%	-	Ylangene
0.03%	-	Isomenthone
0.02%	-	Perillaldehyde
0.02%	-	Bornyl acetate
0.02%	-	alpha-Cubebene
0.02%	-	(E)-beta-Farnesene
0.02%	-	trans-Rose oxide
0.02%	-	Methyl salicylate
0.01%	-	alpha, p-Dimethylstyrene
96.66	TOTAL %	42 COMPOUNDS

Artemisia genipi (Italy)

BOTANICAL SPECIES

Artemisia genipi Weber, fam. Asteraceae (Compositae)

AUTHOR

Mucciarelli, M., Caramiello, R., Maffei, M., and Chialva, F.

TITLE

Essential Oils from Some Artemisia Species Growing Spontaneously in North-West Italy (0.01%= trace)

PUBLICATION

Flavour Fragr. J., Vol. 10, 25-32 (1995)

COMPOUNDS

79.80%	-	alpha-Thujone
10.40%	-	beta-Thujone
1.30%	-	beta-Pinene
1.00%	-	Terpinen-4-ol
0.90%	-	Cuminaldehyde
0.80%	-	alpha-Thujene
0.80%	-	Spathulenol
0.60%	-	para-Cymene
0.60%	-	1, 8-Cineole
0.50%	-	Sabinene
0.50%	-	gamma-Terpinene
0.50%	-	(E)-Nerolidol
0.30%	-	alpha-Pinene
0.30%	-	alpha-Terpinene
0.30%	-	alpha-Terpineol
0.20%	-	Limonene
0.20%	-	Myrtenal

0.20% - Myrtenol

0.20% - Pinocarveol

0.20% - cis-2-Thujenol-4

0.10% - Terpinolene

0.10% - Linalool

0.10% - Borneol

0.10% - Bornyl acetate

0.10% - Pinocarvone

0.01% - Camphene

0.01% - Myrcene

0.01% - alpha-Phellandrene

0.01% - Camphor

0.01% - Carvone

0.01% - beta-Caryophyllene

0.01% - beta-Selinene

0.01% - alpha-Copaene

0.01% - dehydro-1.8-Cineole

0.01% - Yomogi alcohol

0.01% - Artemisia alcohol

0.01% - trans-Verbenol

0.01% - Carvacrol

0.01% - Caryophyllene oxide

0.01% - Sabinene hydrate

0.01% - alpha-Cadinol

0.01% - Verbenone

0.01% - alpha-Fenchene

0.01% - trans-Carveol

0.01% - alpha-Bisabolol

0.01% - Artemisia ketone

0.01% - Artemisyl acetate

0.01% - cis-Chrysanthenyl acetate

0.01%	-	Linalool oxides (cis/trans) (unknown isomers)
0.01%	-	beta-Damascenone
0.01%	-	Ascaridole
0.01%	-	1-epi-Cubenol
0.01%	-	Camphenilone
0.01%	-	Isopinocamphone
0.01%	-	trans-alpha-Bergamotol
0.01%	-	Sabinyl acetate
0.01%	-	trans-Chrysantenyl acetate
0.01%	-	cis-Ocimene epoxide
0.01%	-	Nojigiku alcohol
0.01%	-	Bisabolol oxide (unknown isomer)
100.45		TOTAL % 60 COMPOUNDS

Artemisia glacialis (Italy)

BOTANICAL SPECIES

Artemisia glacialis L., fam. Asteraceae (Compositae)

AUTHOR

Mucciarelii, M., Caramielio, R., Maffei, M., and Chialva, F.

TITLE

Essential Oils from Some Artemisia Species Growing Spontaneously in North-West Italy (0.01% = trace)

PUBLICATION

Flavour Fragr. J., Vol. 10, 25-32 (1995)

COMPOUNDS

31.70%	-	**Camphor**
15.30%	-	**1, 8-Cineole**
9.30%	-	**Spathulenol**
6.40%	-	**Camphene**
6.40%	-	**Caryophyllene oxide**
3.90%	-	**Carvone**
2.90%	-	**alpha-Pinene**
1.80%	-	**beta-Pinene**
1.70%	-	**Terpinen-4-ol**
1.60%	-	**Limonene**
1.60%	-	**Carvacrol**
1.50%	-	**para-Cymene**
1.40%	-	**Sabinyl acetate**
1.30%	-	**Nojigiku alcohol**
1.00%	-	**Cuminaldehyde**
0.90%	-	**alpha-Terpineol**
0.80%	-	**Borneol**

0.80% - Pinocarveol
0.80% - cis-2-Thujenol-4
0.70% - beta-Caryophyllene
0.70% - Sabinene hydrate
0.50% - gamma-Terpinene
0.50% - Verbenone
0.40% - Artemisia alcohol
0.40% - trans-Carveol
0.30% - alpha-Terpinene
0.30% - Myrtenal
0.30% - Pinocarvone
0.30% - Myrtenol
0.20% - Linalool
0.20% - Yomogi alcohol
0.20% - (E)-Nerolidol
0.10% - Terpinolene
0.10% - dehydro-1, 8-Cineole
0.01% - alpha-Thujene
0.01% - Sabinene
0.01% - Myrcene
0.01% - alpha-Phellandrene
0.01% - Bornyl acetate
0.01% - alpha-Copaene
0.01% - alpha-Thujone
0.01% - beta-Thujone
0.01% - trans-Verbenol
0.01% - alpha-Cadinol
0.01% - alpha-Fenchene
0.01% - alpha-Bisabolol
0.01% - Artemisia ketone
0.01% - Artemisyl acetate

0.01%	-	cis-Chrysanthenyl acetate
0.01%	-	Linalool oxides (cis/trans) (unknown isomers)
0.01%	-	beta-Damascenone
0.01%	-	Ascaridole
0.01%	-	gamma-Selinene
0.01%	-	1-epi-Cubenol
0.01%	-	Camphenilone
0.01%	-	Isopinocamphone
0.01%	-	trans-alpha-Bergamotol
0.01%	-	trans-Chrysantenyl acetate
0.01%	-	cis-Ocimene epoxide
0.01%	-	Bisabolol oxide (unknown isomer)
96.56		TOTAL % 60 COMPOUNDS

Artemisia gmelini (Himalaya)

BOTANICAL SPECIES

Artemisia gmelinii Web. ex Stechm., fam. Asteracae (Compositae)

AUTHOR

Mathela, C.S., H. Kharkwal & G.C. Shah

TITLE

Essential Oils Composition of Some Himalayan Artemisia Species

PUBLICATION

J. Essent. Oil Res., Vol. 6, 345 348 (1994)

COMPOUNDS

28.16% - Artemisia ketone
12.96% - 1, 8-Cineole
6.57% - Sabinene
5.13% - Terpinen-4-ol
4.72% - Zingiberene
3.64% - trans-Sabinene hydrate
3.54% - Camphor
2.55% - Cuminaldehyde
2.53% - Germacrene D
1.78% - cis-Sabinene hydrate
1.72% - ar-Curcumene
1.53% - Sabina ketone
1.42% - Yomogi alcohol
1.34% - beta-Caryophyllene
1.02% - para-Cymene
0.69% - alpha-Humulene

0.69%	-	dehydro-1, 8-Cineole	
0.45%	-	Myrtenol	
0.44%	-	alpha-Terpinene	
0.43%	-	beta-Farnesene	
0.34%	-	Isopinocamphone	
0.32%	-	Nonanal	
0.24%	-	Terpinolene	
82.21		TOTAL %	23 COMPOUNDS

Armoise (Morocco)

BOTANICAL SPECIES

Artemisia herba alba Asso, fam. Asteraceae (Compositae)

AUTHOR

Ouyaha, A., R. Negre, J. Viano, Y.F. Lozano & E.M. Gaydou

TITLE

Essential oils from Moroccan Artemisia negrei, A. mesatlantica and A. herbal-alba

PUBLICATION

Lebensmitt. Wiss. u. Technol., Vol. 23, 528-530 (1990)

COMPOUNDS

23.90%	-	alpha-Thujone
20.10%	-	beta-Thujone
14.00%	-	1, 8-Cineole
10.30%	-	Camphor
5.30%	-	alpha-Terpineol
4.20%	-	Chrysanthenone
3.10%	-	alpha-Guaiene
1.80%	-	Camphene
1.70%	-	beta-Elemene
1.50%	-	alpha-Pinene
1.50%	-	gamma-Terpinene
0.80%	-	beta-Pinene
0.80%	-	beta-Caryophyllene
0.70%	-	Borneol
0.20%	-	alpha-Terpinene
0.10%	-	alpha-Thujene
0.10%	-	para-Cymene

0.10%	-	Bornyl acetate
0.10%	-	alpha-Terpinyl acetate
0.10%	-	Artemisia alcohol
0.05%	-	alpha-Humulene
0.05%	-	delta-Cadinene
0.05%	-	gamma-Cadinene
0.05%	-	Thymol
0.05%	-	Myrtenol
0.05 %	-	Carvacrol
0.05%	-	Myrtenyl acetate
0 05%	-	Chrysanthenyl acetate
90.80	TOTAL %	28 COMPOUNDS

Artemisia indica (China)

BOTANICAL SPECIES

Artemisia indica Willd., fam. Asteraceae (Compositae)

AUTHOR

Liangfeng Zhu, Li Yonghua, Li Baoling, Lu Biyao & Xia Nianhe

TITLE

Aromatic Plants and Essential Constituents p. 278

PUBLICATION

South China institute of Botany, Chinese Academy of Sciences, Hai Feng Publishing Co., Chinese National Nodc for APINMAP, distributed by Peace Book Co. Ltd., Hong Kong (1993)

COMPOUNDS

37.27%	-	Artemisia ketone
15.01%	-	1, 8-Cineole
6.97%	-	3, 6, 6-Trimethyl-2-norpinanol
3.67%	-	Camphor
3.00%	-	Borneol
2.83%	-	Piperitol
2.27%	-	2, 4-Dimethyl-2-decene
1.25%	-	alpha-Terpineol
1.13%	-	Terpinen-4-ol
1.01%	-	Piperitone
0.64%	-	7-Octen-4-ol
0.24%	-	Indole
0.23%	-	Nerolidol (unknown isomer)
0.16%	-	beta-Selinene
0.16%	-	Benzaldehyde
75.84	TOTAL %	15 COMPOUNDS

Artemisia judaica (Israel) 1

BOTANICAL SPECIES

Artemisia judaica L. (Bat'aran), fam. Asteraceae (Compositae)

AUTHOR

Fleisher, Z., and Fieisher, A.

TITLE

The Essential Oil of Artemisia judaica L. from the Sinai and Negev Deserts Aromatic Plants of the Holy Land and the Sinai, II (Israeli oil)

PUBLICATION

J. Ess. Oil Res., Vol. 2, 271-273, (Sept./Oct. 1990)

COMPOUNDS

20.96%	-	Artemisia ketone
14.73%	-	Piperitone
13.98%	-	(E)-Ethyl cinnamate
7.80%	-	(Z)-Ethyl cinnamate
5.76%	-	Camphor
4.52%	-	Isophorone
3.01%	-	Artemisia alcohol
2.22%	-	Yomogi alcohol
0.98%	-	Chrysanthenone
0.98%	-	Piperitenone
0.90%	-	1, 3, 5-Trimethylbenzene
0.86%	-	Ethyl isovalerate
0.83%	-	Bornyl acetate
0.76%	-	Filifolone
0.69%	-	Methyl (E)-cinnamate
0.68%	-	Pulegone

0.68% - 1, 2, 4-Trimethyibenzene

0.51% - Borneol

0.51% - Ethyl 3-phenylpropionate

0.49% - 3, 5, 5-Trimethyl-1, 4-cyclohexanedione

0.41% - Methyl (Z)-cinnamate

0.35% - Ethyl phenylacetate

0.32% - para-Cymene

0.24% - (Z)-beta-Ocimene

0.24% - Thymol

0.20% - Santolina alcohol

0.18% - Linalool

0.18% - Cumin alcohol

0.15% - 3-Methyl-3-buten-2-one

0.13% - Benzyl ethyl ether

0.12% - Diosphenol

0.10% - Chrysanthenyl acetate

0.08% - beta-Cadinene

0.07% - alpha-Pinene

0.07% - 1, 8-Cineole

0.07% - Methyl chavicol

0.07% - Acetone

0.06% - Bicyclogermacrene

0.06% - Phenylacetic acid

0.05% - Carvacrol

0.04% - Geranyl acetate

0.04% - Verbenone

0.04% - 2-Methyl-3-butenol-1

0.03% - Tricyclene

0.03% - Camphene

0.03% - Citronellol

0.03% - Germacrene D

0.03%	-	alpha, p-Dimethylstyrene
0.03%	-	Ledene
0.03%	-	cis-Calamenene
0.03%	-	Methyl acetophenone (unknown isomer)
0.03%	-	Davanone
0.03%	-	Propenyl butyrate
0.02%	-	Limonene
0.02%	-	beta-Damascenone
0.02%	-	beta-Ionone
0.02%	-	cis-Jasmone
0.01%	-	cis-Carveol
0.01%	-	Benzyl isovalerate
85.52	TOTAL %	59 COMPOUNDS

Artemisia Judaica (Egypt) 1

BOTANICAL SPECIES

Artemisia judaica L. (Bat'aran), fam. Asteraceae (Compositae)

AUTHOR

Fleisher, Z., and Fieisher, A.

TITLE

The Essential Oil of Artemisia judaica L. from the Sinai and Negev Deserts Aromatic Plants of the Holy Land and the Sinai, II (Egypt: South-Sinai)

PUBLICATION

J. Ess. Oil Res., Vol. 2, 271-273, (Sept./Oct. 1990)

COMPOUNDS

17.53%	-	Piperitone
14.42%	-	Artemisia ketone
9.52%	-	Camphor
6.68%	-	Chrysanthenone
5.56%	-	(E)-Ethyl cinnamate
4.29%	-	(Z)-Ethyl cinnamate
3.25%	-	Artemisia alcohol
2.86%	-	Isophorone
1.53%	-	3, 5, 5-Trimethyl-1, 4-cyclohexanedlone
1.45%	-	Camphene
1.08%	-	Ethyl 2-methylbutyrate
0.99%	-	Bornyl acetate
0.87%	-	Chrysanthenyl acetate
0.77%	-	Yomogi alcohol
0.51%	-	alpha-Pinene
0.46%	-	Ethyl isovalerate

0.40%	-	para-Cymene
0.39%	-	Methyl (E)-cinnamate
0.36%	-	Ethyl phenylacetate
0.32%	-	1, 3, 5-Trimethylbenzene
0.30%	-	Verbenone
0.29%	-	Borneol
0.25%	-	1, 2, 4-Trimethylbenzene
0.24%	-	Ethyl 3-phenylpropionate
0.19%	-	Methyl (Z)-cinnamate
0.18%	-	Filifolone
0.15%	-	Acetone
0.11%	-	Tricyclene
0.11%	-	Limonene
0.11%	-	Piperitenone
0.09%	-	Cumin alcohol
0.08%	-	Nerolidol(unknown isomer)
0.07%	-	Sabinene
0.07%	-	Terpinen-1-ol
0.04%	-	Geranyl acetate
0.04%	-	Santolina alcohol
0.04%	-	Phenylacetic acid
0.03%	-	Thymol
0.03%	-	Sabina ketone
0.02%	-	Myrtenal
0.01%	-	1, 8-Cineole
0.01%	-	Neryl acetate
0.01%	-	Carvacrol
0.01%	-	cis-Jasmone
75.72		TOTAL % 44 COMPOUNDS

Artemisia judaica (Egypt) 2

BOTANICAL SPECIES

Artemisia judaica L. (Bat'aran), fam. Asteraceae (Compositae)

AUTHOR

Fleisher, Z., and Fleisher, A.

TITLE

The Essential Oil of Artemisia judaica L. from the Sinai and Negev Deserts Aromatic Plants of the Holy Land and the Sinai, II (Egypt: Mount-Sinai)

PUBLICATION

J. Ess. Oil Res., Vol. 2, 271-273, (Sept./Oct. 1990)

COMPOUNDS

36.98%	-	Piperitone
13.68%	-	(E)-Ethyl cinnamate
11.53%	-	Camphor
6.84%	-	Chrysanthenone
4.44%	-	(Z)-Ethyl cinnamate
2.43%	-	Bornyl acetate
1.85%	-	Isophorone
1.19%	-	Borneol
0.83%	-	Filifolone
0.61%	-	3, 5, 5-Trimethyl-1, 4-cyclohexanedione
0.54%	-	Decenoic acid (unknown isomer)
0.51%	-	Thymol
0.47%	-	1, 3, 5-Trimethylbenzene
0.46%	-	1, 2, 4-Trimethylbenzene
0.42%	-	Ethyl 2-methylbutyrate
0.33%	-	para-Cymene

0.32%	-	Diosphenol
0.32%	-	Ethyl phenylacetate
0.30%	-	Methyl (E)-cinnamate
0.28%	-	Linalool
0.28%	-	Ethyl isovalerate
0.27%	-	Carvacrol
0.25%	-	Chrysanthenyl acetate
0.21%	-	Ethyl 3-phenylpropionate
0.19%	-	Cumin alcohol
0.18%	-	Piperitenone
0.16%	-	Nerolidol (unknown isomer)
0.15%	-	Camphene
0.13%	-	1, 8-Cineole
0.11%	-	alpha-Terpineol
0.11%	-	Verbenone
0.11%	-	Terpinen-1-ol
0.10%	-	Germacrene D
0.09%	-	Methyl (Z)-cinnamate
0.08%	-	Limonene
0.07%	-	Geranyl acetate
0.06%	-	cis-Carveol
0.04%	-	beta-Cadinene
0.04%	-	Viridiflorol
0.03%	-	Pinocarvone
0.03%	-	beta-Damascenone
0.03%	-	cis-Jasmone
0.03%	-	Ethyl octanoate
0.02%	-	beta-Ionone
0.02%	-	Benzyl isovalerate
87.12	TOTAL %	45 COMPOUNDS

Artemisia judaica (Israel) 2

BOTANICAL SPECIES

Artemisia judaica L., fam. Asteraceae (Compositae)

AUTHOR

Ravid, U., et al.

TITLE

The Essentiai Oil of Artemisia Judaica L. Chemotypes (average concentrations of 6 samples from Israel (Negev) and Sinai)

PUBLICATION

Flavour Fragr. J, Vol. 7, 69-72 (1992)

COMPOUNDS

16.50%	-	Piperitone
13.50%	-	Artemisia ketone
10.50%	-	Camphor
7.50%	-	Artemisia alcohol
6.50%	-	(E)-Ethyl cinnamate
6.30%	-	Chrysanthenone
4.80%	-	2, 2, 6-Trimethylcyclohex-5-enone
3.00%	-	Yomogi alcohol
3.00%	-	Filifolide 2
2.50%	-	(Z)-Ethyl cinnamate
1.90%	-	Borneol
1.50%	-	Bornyl acetate
1.50%	-	Artemisyl acetate
1.10%	-	Filifolide 1
0.70%	-	Chrysanthenyl acetate
0.65%	-	Linalool
0.60%	-	Camphene

0.60% - 3, 5, 5-Trimethyl-2-cyclohexene-1, 4-dione
0.60% - Filifolone
0.50% - Verbenone
0.45% - Davanone
0.40% - Guaiol
0 40% - Methyl (E)-cinnamate
0.30% - para-Cymene
0.30% - Terpinen-4-ol
0.30% - Ethyl 2-methylbutyrate
0.30% - Ethyl isovalerate
0 30% - Propyl isovalerate
0.25% - Bicyclogermacrene
0.25% - (Z)-Methyl jasmonate
0.25% - trans-Chrysanthenol
0.20% - Carvone
0.20% - alpha-Cubebene
0.15% - Tricyclene
0.15% - delta-3-Carene
0.15% - alpha-Terpineol
0.15% - p-Cymen-8-ol
0.15% - Santolina alcohol
0.15% - Ethyl phenylacetate
0.15% - Ethyl 3-phenylpropionate
0.15% - Artemisiatriene
0.15% - Propyl phenylacetate
0.10% - Sabinene
0.10% - Myrcene
0.10% - Geranyl acetate
0.10% - Thymol
0.10% - Carvacrol
0.10% - (E)-Nerolidol

0.10%	-	Germacrene D
0.10%	-	Methyl (Z)-cinnamate
0.10%	-	Decanoic acid
0.10%	-	nor-Davanone
0.10%	-	Propyl 2-methylbutyrate
0.05%	-	alpha-Pinene
0.05%	-	Limonene
0.05%	-	(E)-Anethole
0.03%	-	Viridiflorol
0.03%	-	Guaiyl acetate
0.01%	-	alpha-Phellandrene
0.01%	-	gamma-Terpinene
0.01%	-	delta-Cadinene
90.34		TOTAL % 61 COMPOUNDS

Artemisia kawakamii (China)

BOTANICAL SPECIES

Artemisia kawakamii Hayata, fam. Asteraceae (Compositae)

AUTHOR

Liangfeng Zhu, Li Yonghua, Li Baoling, Lu Biyao & Xia Nianhe

TITLE

Aromatic Plants and Essential Constituents p. 279

PUBLICATION

South China Institute of Botany, Chinese Academy of Sciences, Hai Feng Publishing Co., Chinese National Node for APINMAP, distributed by Peace Book Co. Ltd., Hong Kong (1993).

COMPOUNDS

26.23%	-	Camphor
14.73%	-	trans-Sabinol
7.44%	-	cis-Sabinol
5.69%	-	Borneol
2.14%	-	Carveol
1.82%	-	Carvyl acetate
1.02%	-	Methyl isoeugenol
1.00%	-	Linalool
0.91%	-	alpha-Terpineol
0.86%	-	delta-Cadinol
0.84%	-	Terpinen-4-ol
0.66%	-	Isoborneol
0.64%	-	alpha-Curcumene
0.43%	-	Bornyl acetate
0.43%	-	6-Methyl-5-hepten-2-one
0.37%	-	Guaiol
0.32%	-	Myrtenol
0.30%	-	Eugenol
65.83	TOTAL %	18 COMPOUNDS

Artemisia macrocephala (China)

BOTANICAL SPECIES

Artemisia macrocephala Jacq. ex Bess., fam. Asteraceae (Compositae)

AUTHOR

Liangfeng Zhu, Li Yonghua, Li Baoling, Lu Biyao & Xia Nianhe

TITLE

Aromatic Plants and Essential Constituents p. 280

PUBLICATION

South China institute of Botany, Chinese Academy of Sciences, Hai Feng Publishing Co., Chinese National Node for APINMAP, distributed by Peace Book Co. Ltd., Hong Kong (1993)

COMPOUNDS

38.36%	-	1, 8-Cineole
5.58%	-	Borneol
4.73%	-	Geranyl 2-methyibutyrate
4.10%	-	Linalool
3.89%	-	alpha-Terpineol
3.35%	-	Terpinen-4-ol
3.09%	-	Methyl 2,4-hexadienoate
2.99%	-	Phenylacetonitrile
2.45%	-	Camphor
2.44%	-	Geranyl 2, 2-dimethylpropionate
1.37%	-	Nonanal
1.19%	-	2-Methylhexanoic acid
1.05%	-	Pentanoic acid
0.97%	-	Azulene
0.12%	-	alpha-Thujone
75.68	TOTAL %	15 COMPOUNDS

Artemisia maritima (Himalaya)

BOTANICAL SPECIES

Artemisia maritima L., fam. Asteraceae (Compositae)

AUTHOR

Mathela, C.S., H. Kharkwal & G.C. Shah

TITLE

Essential Oil Composition of Some Himalyan Artemisia Species

PUBLICATION

J. Essent. Oil Res., Vol. 6, 345-348 (1994)

COMPOUNDS

63.25%	-	alpha-Thujone
7.83%	-	Sabinene
6.54%	-	1, 8-Cineole
2.22%	-	Germacrene D
1.14%	-	Terpinen-4-ol
1.00%	-	beta-Caryophyllene
0.83%	-	Cuminaldehyde
0.68%	-	para-Cymene
0.67%	-	Sabina ketone
0.54%	-	trans-Sabinene hydrate
0.54%	-	Isopinocamphone
0.42%	-	cis-Sabinene hydrate
0.23%	-	alpha-Terpinene
85.89	TOTAL %	13 COMPOUNDS

Artemisia molinieri

BOTANICAL SPECIES

Artemisia molinieri Quezel, Barbero et R. Loisel, Asteraceae (Compos)

AUTHOR

Carnat, A. -P. and Lamaison, J. -L.

TITLE

Composition of the Essential Oil of Artemisia molinieri Quezel, Barbero et R. Loisel

PUBLICATION

J. Essent, Oil Res., Vol. 4, 635-637 (Nov/Dcc 1992)

COMPOUNDS

62.12%	-	Ascaridole
12.22%	-	para-Cymene
9.56%	-	alpha-Terpinene
1.78%	-	Germacrene D
1.74%	-	1, 8-Cineole
0.59%	-	gamma-Terpinene
0.45%	-	Terpinen-4-ol
0.35%	-	Cumin alcohol
0.31%	-	cis-Jasmone
0.28%	-	Carvacrol
0.28%	-	alpha-Bisabolol
0.26%	-	Sabinene
0.23%	-	cis-p-Menth-2-en-1-ol
0.20%	-	Eugenol
0.18%	-	Thymol
0.18%	-	trans-p-Menth-2-en-1-ol

0.11%	-	Limonene	
0.08%	-	Camphene	
0.06%	-	alpha-Pinene	
0.04%	-	Myrcene	
91.02		TOTAL %	20 COMPOUNDS

Artemisia monosperma

BOTANICAL SPECIES

Artemisia monosperma Del., fam. Asteraceae (Compositae)

AUTHOR

Hifnawy, M.S., Abdel Wahab, S.M., El-Hawary, S.S., and Karawya, M.S.

TITLE

Study of Essential Oil of Artemisia monosperma Del. and its Larvicidal Effect

PUBLICATION

In: Proceedings 11th intern. Congress of Essential Oils, Fragrances and Flavours, 12-16 Nov., 1989, New Delhi, India, Vol. 4, 55-61

COMPOUNDS

36.00%	-	Dibenzofuran
25.00%	-	1-Phenylbicyclo [3.3.1]non-2-en-9-ol
12.00%	-	Phenanthrene, octahydro-
4.00%	-	Diphenyl
4.00%	-	(Z)-3-Heptenal
3.00%	-	Isooctyl phthalate
2.00%	-	Diphenylamine
2.00%	-	1-Ethyl-3, 5-di(isopropyl)benzene
2.00%	-	Tetra ethylbenzene
1.00%	-	Ethyl benzoate
0.50%	-	Artemisia ketone
0.50%	-	Sesquiterpene alcohols (unknown)
0.50%	-	Tricyclo [7.5.0.0.(4,8)] tetradeca-1 (9),2,4(8) triene
0.50%	-	(E)-Tagetone

0.30%	-	3-Heptenal
0.20%	-	trans-beta-Bergamotene
0.20%	-	4-Cyclohexyicyciohexanol
0.20%	-	1, 2-Dimethyl-3-ethylbenzene
0.10%	-	Camphor
0.10%	-	Farnesol (unknown isomer)
0.10%	-	Isopropylcyclohexane
0.10%	-	2-Ethylhexanol
0.10%	-	2-(2-Butynyl)-cyclohexanone
94.40	TOTAL %	23 COMPOUNDS

Artemisia moorcroftiana

BOTANICAL SPECIES

Artemisia moorcroftiana, fam. Asteraceae (Compositae)

AUTHOR

Weyerstahl, P.

TITLE

New Constituents from Some North-West Indian Artemisia Oils: Anaiysis and Synthesis

PUBLICATION

Newer Trends in Essential Oils and Flavours p. 26, K.L. Dhar, R.K. Thappa, S.G. Agarwal Eds., Tata McGrawe-Hili Publ. Co. Ltd., New Dehii (1993)

COMPOUNDS

12.80%	-	alpha-Thujone
10.20%	-	Artemisia ketone
7.70%	-	beta-Pinene
5.80%	-	1, 8-Cineole
5.40%	-	Camphor
4.00%	-	beta-Thujone
3.30%	-	Sabinene
2.60%	-	alpha-Pinene
2.60%	-	Terpinen-4-ol
2.60%	-	(E)-Nerolidol
2.60%	-	Vulgarone B
2.50%	-	Piperitone
2.50%	-	Artemisia alcohol
2 30%	-	Germacrene D
2.20%	-	Borneol
2.10%	-	3-exo-Acetoxybornyl acetate

1.80%	-	Camphene
1.80%	-	Yomogi alcohol
1.50%	-	Myrtenol
1.40%	-	cis-Chrysanthenol
1.40%	-	alpha-Longipinen-7beta-ol
1.20%	-	Myrtenal
1.10%	-	para-Cymene
1.10%	-	trans-p-Menth-2-en-1-ol
1.00%	-	Bicyclogermacrene
0.88%	-	Bornyl acetate
0.88%	-	trans-Sabinene hydrate
0 80%	-	Spathulenol
0.75%	-	trans-Pinocarveol
0.65%	-	cis-Chrysanthenyl acetate
0.63%	-	gamma-Terpinene
0.60%	-	Limonene
0.60%	-	cis-Sabinene hydrate
0.56%	-	Pinocarvone
0.50%	-	alpha-Longipinene
0.44%	-	cis-Piperitol
0.42%	-	trans-Verbenol
0.40%	-	3-exo-Hydroxybornyl acetate
0.39%	-	delta-Terpineol
0.37%	-	alpha-Terpineol
0.36%	-	Eremoligenol
0.34%	-	Myrcene
0.34%	-	Caryophyllene oxide
0.26%	-	neo-Thujanol-3
0.24%	-	alpha-Terpinene
0.21%	-	Terpinolene
0.20%	-	trans-alpha-Bergamotene

0.18%	-	Davanone	
0.17%	-	alpha-Thujene	
0.16%	-	alpha-Cadinol	
0.16%	-	allo-Aromadendrene	
0.14%	-	alpha-Phellandrene	
0.13%	-	Cuminaldehyde	
0.12%	-	H-Selinenol-4,alpha	
0.10%	-	beta-Eudesmol	
0.10%	-	gamma-Decalactone	
0.10%	-	3-exo-Acetoxy-borneol	
0.06%	-	gamma-Nonalactone	
0.01%	-	alpha-Cubebene	
0.01%	-	Sabina ketone	
0.01%	-	cis-p-Menth-2-en-1-ol	
95.77		TOTAL %	61 COMPOUNDS

Artemisia nilagirica (vulgaris) (India) 2

BOTANICAL SPECIES

Artemisia nilagirica (C.B. Clarks) Pamp. (A. vulgaris Hook f.), Asteraceae

AUTHOR

Thakur, R.S., and Misra, L.N.

TITLE

Essential Oils of Indian Artemisia (Nilgiri chemotype)

PUBLICATION

In: Proceedings 11th Intern. Congress of Essential Oils, Fragrances and Flavours, 12-16 Nov., 1989, New Delhi, India Vol. 4, 127-135.

COMPOUNDS

56.30%	-	alpha-Thujone
7.49%	-	beta-Thujone
3.30%	-	para-Cymene
3.01%	-	Camphor
2.21%	-	beta-Pinene
2.21%	-	alpha-Terpineol
1.53%	-	Geraniol
1.51%	-	beta-Caryophyllene
1.17%	-	gamma-Cadinene
1.14%	-	Linalool
0.92%	-	Eugenol
0.53%	-	Limonene
0.45%	-	Camphene
0.27%	-	alpha-Pinene
0.01%	-	alpha-Thujene
0.01%	-	Sabinene

0.01%	-	Myrcene	
0.01%	-	Terpinolene	
0.01%	-	Borneol	
0.01%	-	Bornyl acetate	
0.01%	-	Aromadendrene	
82.11		TOTAL %	21 COMPOUNDS

Artemisia nilagirica (vulgaris) (India) 1

BOTANICAL SPECIES

Artemisia nilagirica (C.B.Clarks) Pamp. (A. vulgaris Hook f.), Asteraceae

AUTHOR

Thakur, R.S., and Misra L.N.

TITLE

Essential Oils of Indian Artemisia (A. nilagirica syn. A. vulgaris, North Indian chemotype)

PUBLICATION

in: Proceedings 11th Intern. Congress of Essential Oils, Fragrances and Flavours, 12-16 Nov., 1989, New Delhi, India, vol. 4, 127-135

COMPOUNDS

20.00% - Sesquiterpene alcohols (unknown)
9.74% - Camphor
7.98% - beta-Eudesmol
657% - 1, 8-Cineole
3.41% - Artemisia alcohol
2.59% - Camphene
1.92% - alpha-Gurjunene
1.62% - alpha-Eudesmol
1.60% - para-Cymene
1.35% - cis-alpha-Santalol
1.24% - Terpinen-4-ol
1.20% - alpha-Pinene
0.96% - cis-Alloocimene
0.90% - Bornyl acetate
0.59% - Linalool oxides (cis/trans) (unknown isomers)

0.58%	-	alpha-Tnujone	
0.56%	-	beta-Pinene	
0.54%	-	Linalyl acetate	
0.42%	-	Phellandral	
0.31%	-	beta-Caryophyllene	
0.27%	-	7-Octenol-1	
0.23%	-	beta-Thujone	
0.22%	-	Sabinene	
0.21%	-	trans-Alloocimene	
0.10%	-	gamma-Terpinene	
0.09%	-	alpha-Thujene	
65.20		TOTAL %	26 COMPOUNDS

Artemisia occidentalis-sichaunensis (China)

BOTANICAL SPECIES

Artemisia occidentalis-sichuanensis Y.R. Ling et S.Y. Zhao, fam. Asteraceae

AUTHOR

Liangfeng Zhu, Li Yonghua, Li Baoling, Lu Biyao & Xia Nianhe

TITLE

Aromatic Plants and Essential Constituents p. 281

PUBLICATION

South China Institute of Botany, Chinese Academy of Sciences, Hai Feng Publishing Co., Chinese National Node for APINMAP, distributed by Peace Book Co. Ltd., Hong Kong (1993)

COMPOUNDS

11.10%	-	Borneol
7.06%	-	1, 8-Cineole
6.41%	-	beta-Cubebene
5.85%	-	Sabinene
5.02%	-	beta-Caryophyllene
4.16%	-	Linalool
3.84%	-	Camphor
3.13%	-	7-Octen-4-ol
2.70%	-	beta-Farnesene
2.19%	-	alpha-Terpineol
2.09%	-	beta-Cadinene
2.01%	-	Piperitol
1.80%	-	Terpinen-4-ol
1.66%	-	Eremophllene
1.17%	-	para-Cymene

1.06%	-	Guaiol	
0.90%	-	delta-Cadinol	
0.85%	-	Zingiberene	
0.75%	-	Copaene (unknown isomer)	
0.73%	-	gamma-Cadinene	
0.64%	-	6-Methyl-5-hepten-2-one	
0.64%	-	Artemisiatriene	
0.43%	-	alpha-Phellandrene	
0.34%	-	3-Octanol	
0.33%	-	Myrtenol	
0.32%	-	alpha-Pinene	
0.25%	-	2-Hexenal	
0.20%	-	Eugenol	
0.19%	-	gamma-Terpinene	
0.18%	-	Octyl acetate	
0.17%	-	Perillaldehyde	
0.17%	-	Piperitone	
68.34		TOTAL %	32 COMPOUNDS

Davana 1

BOTANICAL SPECIES

Artemisia pallens Wall. ex DC., fam. Asteraceae (Compositae)

AUTHOR

Klimes, I., and Lamparsky, D.

TITLE

Analytical results concerning the essential oil of Artemisia pallens (Wall.)

PUBLICATION

Progress in Essential Oils, E.-J. Brunke Ed., Walter de Gruyter & Co., Berlin p. 197-214(1986)

COMPOUNDS

66.30%	-	Davanone
6.00%	-	Bicyclogermacrene
3.40%	-	Spathulenol
3.00%	-	5-Ethenyldihydro-5-methyl-2(3H)-furanone
2.90%	-	T-Cadinol
2.00%	-	beta-Eudesmol
0.50%	-	allo-Aromadendrene
0.30%	-	Linalool
0.30%	-	Bicycloelemene
0.23%	-	Aromadendrene
0.20%	-	beta-Cubebene
0.20%	-	beta-Maaliene
0.10%	-	Lavender lactol
0.10%	-	Selin-6-en-11-ol
0.05%	-	trans-Linalool oxide (5) (furanoid)
0.05%	-	cis-Linalool oxide (5) (furanoid)
0.01%	-	alpha-Gurjunene
0.01%	-	Ledene
85.65	TOTAL %	18 COMPOUNDS

Davana (India) 1

BOTANICAL SPECIES

Artemisia pallens Wall. ex DC., fam. Asteraceae (Compositae)

AUTHOR

Thakur, R.S. and Misra, L.N.,

TITLE

Essential Oils of Indian Artemisia

PUBLICATION

In: Proceedings 11th Intern. Congress of Essential Oils, Fragrances and Flavours, 12-16 Nov., 1989, New Delhi, India, Vol. 4, 127-135

COMPOUNDS

55.00%	-	Davanone
10.00%	-	Nerol
5.00%	-	Geraniol
3.00%	-	Davanone, hydroxy-
2.50%	-	dihydro-Rosefurans
2.00%	-	Furano-nordeterpenoid
2.00%	-	Hydroxy-necolidol
1.50%	-	Davana ethers
1.50%	-	Artemone
1.00%	-	Lavender lactol
1.00%	-	Davanafurans
0.50%	-	Hydroxydihydrorosefuran
0.05%	-	Camphene
0.05%	-	Sabinene
0.05%	-	para-Cymene
0.05%	-	Linalool

0.05%	-	Borneol
0.05%	-	gamma-Cadinene
0.05%	-	Eugenol
0.05%	-	Farnesol (unknown isomer)
0.05%	-	Methyl eugenol
0.05%	-	Linalool oxides (cis/trans) (unknown isomers)
0.05%	-	Methyl isoeugenol
0.05%	-	Lilac aldehyde
0.05%	-	nor-Davanone
0.05%	-	Lilac alcohol
85.70	TOTAL %	26 COMPOUNDS

Davana (India) 2

BOTANICAL SPECIES

Artemisia pallens Wall. ex DC., fam. Asteraceae (Compositae)

AUTHOR

Misra J.N., Chandra A. and Thakur R.S.

TITLE

Fragrant components of oil from Artemisia pallens

PUBLICATION

Phytochemistry, Vol. 30, 549-552 (1991)

COMPOUNDS

38.00%	-	cis-Davanone
10.00%	-	Nerol
5.00%	-	Geraniol
5.00%	-	trans-Davanone
3.00%	-	iso-Davanone
3.00%	-	Davanone, cis-hydroxy-
2.50%	-	Davanic acid
2.00%	-	Cinnamyl cinnamate
2.00%	-	Davanone, trans-hydroxy-
2.00%	-	11 -Hydroxy-8-oxo-9,10-dehydro-10,11 dihydronerolidol
1.50%	-	Sesquiterpene alcohols (unknown)
1.50%	-	Davana ethers
1.50%	-	Artemone
1.50%	-	nor-Davanone
1.50%	-	2alpha-(3-Methylbut-2-enyl)-4-methyl-2,5 dihydrofuran
1.00%	-	trans-Davanafuran

1.00%	-	2beta-(3-Methylbut-2-enyl)-4-methyl-2,5 dihydrofuran
0.80%	-	para-Cymene
0.80%	-	gamma-Cadinene
0.80%	-	Davanol
0.70%	-	Ethyl davanate
0.50%	-	Linalool
0.50%	-	Bomeol
0.50%	-	Farnesol (unknown isomer)
0.50%	-	Linalool oxides (cis/trans) (unknown isomers)
0.50%	-	Lilac aldehyde
0.50%	-	Lilac alcohol
0.50%	-	cis-Davanafuran
0.50%	-	Rosefuran, hydroxydihydro-
0.50%	-	8-Oxonerolidol
0.05%	-	Camphene
0.05%	-	Sabinene
0.05%	-	nor-Davana ether
89.75	TOTAL %	33 COMPOUNDS

Artemisia persica (India)

BOTANICAL SPECIES

Artemisia persica Boiss., fam. Asteraceae (Compositae)

AUTHOR

Weyerstahl, P., and Marschall-Weyerstahl, H., & Kaul, V.K.

TITLE

Constituents of the Essential Oil of Artemisia persica

PUBLICATION

J. Ess. Oil Res., Vol. 4, 1-7 (Jan./Feb. 1992)

COMPOUNDS

23.60%	-	Artemisia ketone
7.00%	-	trans-Sabinol
6.30%	-	Sabinyl acetate
5.90%	-	Sabinene
5.20%	-	1, 8-Ciheole
5.20%	-	alpha-Tnujone
4.80%	-	Terpinen-4-ol
4.70%	-	Yomogi alcohol
2.20%	-	Dehydrosabina ketone
1.90%	-	gamma-Terpinene
1.70%	-	Artemisyl acetate
1.70%	-	Sabina ketone
1.60%	-	Artemisia alcohol
1.40%	-	ar-Curcumene
1.40%	-	Cuminaldehyde
1.40%	-	Zingiberene
1.40%	-	p-Menth-2-en-l-ol
1.30%	-	trans-Sabinene hydrate

1.30%	-	cis-Sabinene hydrate
1.10%	-	para-Cymene
1.10%	-	beta-Thujone
1.10%	-	Artedouglasia oxide A
1.00%	-	alpha-Terpinene
0.90%	-	Artedouglasia oxide C
0.86%	-	Thuj-3-en-I0-al
0.70%	-	dehydro-1, 8-Cineole
0.68%	-	alpha-Terpineol
0.53%	-	Cumin alcohol
0.48%	-	Vulgarone B
0.43%	-	Terpinolene
0.42%	-	Artedouglasia oxide D
0.42%	-	Artedouglasia oxide B
0.40%	-	Camphor
0.40%	-	beta-Bisabolene
0.31%	-	p-Mentha-1, 3-dien-7-al
0.30%	-	Myrtenol
0.28%	-	(E)-beta-Farnesene
0.25%	-	Germacrene D
0.25%	-	Laciniatafuranone H
0.20%	-	alpha-Thujene
0.20%	-	(Z)-beta-Farnesene
0.19%	-	Spathulenol
0.14%	-	alpha-Pinene
0.14%	-	Myrtenal
0.11%	-	beta-Pinene
0.10%	-	Artemisiatriene
0.10%	-	Laciniatafuranone, isomer
0.08%	-	Davanone
93.17		TOTAL % 48 COMPOUNDS

Artemisia petrosa (Italy)

BOTANICAL SPECIES

Artemisia petrosa Baumg. ssp. eriantha Ten., fam. Asteraceae (Compositae)

AUTHOR

Mucciarelli, M., Caramiello, R., Maffei, M., and Chialva, F.

TITLE

Essential Oils from Some Artemisia Species Growing Spontaneously in North-West Italy

PUBLICATION

Flavour Fragr. J, Vol. 10, 25-32 (1995)

COMPOUNDS

69.70%	-	alpha-Thujone
16.80%	-	beta-Thujone
4.10%	-	Spathulenol
0.90%	-	trans-Pinocarveol
0.70%	-	Cuminaldehyde
0.60%	-	1, 8-Cineole
0.60%	-	alpha-Fenchene
0.60%	-	Sabinyl acetate
0.50%	-	para-Cymene
0.30%	-	alpha-Pinene
0.30%	-	beta-Pinene
0.30%	-	Terpinen-4-ol
0.30%	-	Carvacrol
0.30%	-	Caryophyllene oxide
0.20%	-	Sabinene
0.20%	-	Limonene

0.20% - Borneol
0.20% - alpha-Terpineol
0.20% - Myrtenol
0.20% - Ascaridole
0.10% - alpha-Thujene
0.10% - gamma-Terpinene
0.10% - Pinocarvone
0.10% - Linalool oxides (cis/trans) (unknown isomers)
0.10% - cis-2-Thujenol-4
0.01% - Camphene
0.01% - Myrcene
0.01% - alpha-Phellandrene
0.01% - alpha-Terpinene
0.01% - Terpinolene
0.01% - Linalool
0.01% - Camphor
0.01% - Carvone
0.01% - Bornyl acetate
0.01% - beta-Caryophyllene
0.01% - alpha-Copaene
0.01% - Myrtenal
0.01% - dehydro-1, 8-Cineole
0.01% - Yomogi alcohol
0.01% - Artemisia alcohol
0.01% - trans-Verbenol
0.01% - Sabinene hydrate
0.01% - (E)-Nerolidol
0.01% - alpha-Cadinol
0.01% - Verbenone
0.01% - trans-Carveol

0.01%	-	alpha-Bisabolol	
0.01%	-	Artemisia ketone	
0.01%	-	Artemisyl acetate	
0.01%	-	cis-Chrysanthenyl acetate	
0.01%	-	beta-Damascenone	
0.01%	-	gamma-Selinene	
0.01%	-	1-epi-Cubenol	
0.01%	-	Camphenilone	
0.01%	-	Isopinocamphone	
0.01%	-	trans-alpha-Bergamotol	
0.01%	-	trans-Chrysantenyl acetate	
0.01%	-	cis-Ocimene epoxide	
0.01%	-	Nojigiku alcohol	
0.01%	-	Bisabolol oxide (unknown isomer)	
98.05		TOTAL %	60 COMPOUNDS

Wormwood Roman, headspace

BOTANICAL SPECIES

Artemisia pontica L, fam. Aste.raceae (Compositae)

AUTHOR

Chialva, F., Gabri, G., Liddle, P.A.P., and Ulian, F.

TITLE

Qualitative Evaluation of Aromatic Herbs by Direct Headspace GC Analysis. Applications of the Method and Comparison with the Trad. Analysis of E.O.

PUBLICATION

Journal of HRC & CC, Vol. 5, April 1982, 182-188

COMPOUNDS

46.00%	-	Artemisia ketone
22.80%	-	1, 8-Cineole
14.30%	-	alpha-Thujone
1.80%	-	beta-Thujone
0.20%	-	alpha-Pinene
0.05%	-	Sabinene
0.05%	-	beta-Pinene
0.05%	-	Myrcene
0.05%	-	alpha-Phellandrene
0.05%	-	para-Cymene
0.05%	-	Limonene
0.05%	-	garnma-Terpinene
0.05%	-	Hotrienol
85.50	TOTAL %	13 COMPOUNDS

Wormwood Roman

BOTANICAL SPECIES

Artemisia pontica L., fam. Asteraceae (Compositae)

AUTHOR

Chialva, F., Gabri, G., Liddle, P.A.P. and Ulian, F.

TITLE

Qualitative Evaluation of Aromatic Herbs by Direct Headspace GC Analysis. Applications of the Method and Comparison with the Trad. Analysis of E.O.

PUBLICATION

Journ. of HRC & CC, Vol. 5, April 1982, 182-188

COMPOUNDS

22.80%	-	Artemisia ketone
13.50%	-	alpha-Thujone
13.00%	-	1, 8-Cineole
3.30%	-	beta-Thujone
2.90%	-	Limonene
1.90%	-	Caryophyllene oxide
1.90%	-	Pontica epoxide
1.60%	-	Hotrienol
1.40%	-	gamma-Cadinene
1.30%	-	para-Cymene
1.00%	-	beta-Caryophyllene
0.70%	-	gamma-Terpinene
0.60%	-	Thymol
0.60%	-	Sesquiterpene alcohols (unknown)
0.50%	-	beta-Bourbonene
0.40%	-	alpha-Copaene

0.20%	-	Carvacrol
0.10%	-	alpha-Pinene
0.10%	-	Eugenol
0.05%	-	Sabinene
0.05%	-	beta-Pinene
0.05%	-	Myrcene
0.05%	-	Geraniol
68.00	TOTAL %	23 COMPOUNDS

Artemisia princeps (China)

BOTANICAL SPECIES

Artemisia princeps Pamp., fam. Asteraceae (Compositae)

AUTHOR

Liangfeng Zhu, Li Yonghua, Li Baoling, Lu Biyao & Xia Nianhe

TITLE

Aromatic Plants and Essential Constituents p. 282

PUBLICATION

South China Institute of Botany, Chinese Academy of Sciences, Hai Feng Publishing Co., Chinese National Node for APINMAP, distributed by Peace Book Co. Ltd., Hong Kong (1993).

COMPOUNDS

11.18%	-	beta-Caryophyllene
8.60%	-	1, 8-Cineole
6.93%	-	Camphor
5.10%	-	7-Octen-4-ol
4.02%	-	alpha-Humulene
2.48%	-	beta-Cubebene
2.37%	-	Artemisia ketone
2.28%	-	Borneol
2.26%	-	Cadinol (unknown structure)
2.02%	-	Myrtenol
1.63%	-	beta-Selinene
1.41%	-	allo-Aromadendrene
1.38%	-	Pinocarveol
1.22%	-	alpha-Curcumene
1.17%	-	2-Hexenal
0.89%	-	Linalool

0.75%	-	beta-Elemene
0.75%	-	2, 3-Dihydrobenzofuran
0.72%	-	Eugenol
0.57%	-	Terpinen-4-ol
0.45%	-	Hexanal
0.45%	-	Propylcyclopropane
0.35%	-	alpha-Elemene
0.33%	-	Phenylacetaldehyde
0.27%	-	Benzaldehyde
0.26%	-	2-Phenylethanol
0.24%	-	alpha-Pinene
0.22%	-	Furfural
60.30	TOTAL %	28 COMPOUNDS

Artemisia pubescens (China)

BOTANICAL SPECIES

Artemisia pubescens Ledeb., fam. Asteraceae (Labiatae)

AUTHOR

Liangfeng Zhu, Li Yonghua, Li Baoling, Lu Biyao & Xia Nianhe

TITLE

Aromatic Plants and Essential Constituents p. 283

PUBLICATION

South China Institute of Botany, Chinese Academy of Sciences, Hai Feng Publishing Co., Chinese National Node for APINMAP, distributed by Peace Book Co. Ltd., Hong Kong (1993)

COMPOUNDS

53.31%	-	Capillene
2.17%	-	iso-Capillene
1.35%	-	Eremophilene
1.20%	-	alpha-Curcumene
1.15%	-	Bornyl acetate
1.04%	-	1, 8-Cineole
0.98%	-	Terpinen-4-ol
0.85%	-	Borneol
0.70%	-	Coumarin
0.51%	-	alpha-Humulene
0.48%	-	alpha-Terpineol
0.46%	-	Carveol
0.45%	-	Linalool
64.68	TOTAL %	13 COMPOUNDS

Artemisia roburghiana (Himalaya)

BOTANICAL SPECIES

Artemisia roxburghiana Wall. ex Bies, var. hypolenca, fam. Asteraceae

AUTHOR

Mathela, C.S., H. Kharkwal & G.C. Shah

TITLE

Essential Oil Composition of Some Himalayan Artemisia Species (0.01% = trace)

PUBLICATION

J. Essent. Oil Res., Vol. 6, 345-348 (1994)

COMPOUNDS

65.30%	-	beta-Thujone
3.30%	-	alpha-Thujone
3.00%	-	Sabina ketone
2.80%	-	beta-Caryophyllene
2.80%	-	trans-Sabinene hydrate
2.50%	-	Lavandulyl acetate
2.00%	-	Terpinen-4-ol
1.50%	-	Thujyl acetate
1.30%	-	para-Cymene
1.10%	-	Sabinene
1.00%	-	1, 8-Cineole
1.00%	-	Germacrene D
0.20%	-	Bicyclogennacrene
0.10%	-	Spathulenol
0.10%	-	Caryophyllene oxide
0.10%	-	trans-alpha-Bergamotene

0.01%	-	Myrcene
0.01%	-	Limonene
0.01%	-	gamma-Terpinene
0.01%	-	Terpinolene
0.01%	-	Nonanal
0.01%	-	Linalool
0.01%	-	alpha-Copaene
0.01%	-	Myrtenol
0.01%	-	Eugenol
0.01%	-	alpha-Gurjunene
0.01%	-	T-Cadinol
0.01%	-	T-Muurolol
0.01%	-	alpha-Cadinol
0.01%	-	6-Methyl-5-hepten-2-one
0.01%	-	Hotrienol
0.01%	-	Lavandulol
0.01%	-	Cubebol
0.01%	-	cis-Pinocarveol
0.01%	-	cis-Sabinyl acetate
0.01%	-	Seychellene
88.30		TOTAL % 36 COMPOUNDS

Artemisia scoparia (India)

BOTANICAL SPECIES

Artemisia scoparia Waldst. & Kit., fam. Asteraceae (Compositae)

AUTHOR

Thakur, R.S., and Misra, L.N.

TITLE

Essential Oils of Indian Artemisia

PUBLICATION

In: Proceedings 11th intern. Congress of Essential Oils, Fragrances and Flavours, 12-16 Nov., 1989, New Delhi, India, Vol. 4, 127-135

COMPOUNDS

30.00%	-	Eugenol
15.00%	-	Agropinene
0.05%	-	alpha-Pinene
0.05%	-	beta-Pinene
0.05%	-	Carvone
0.05%	-	Geranyl acetate
0.05%	-	beta-Caryophyllene
0.05%	-	gamma-Cadinene
0.05%	-	Caryophyllene oxide
0.05%	-	Butanal
0.05%	-	Methyl heptenone (unknown structure)
0.05%	-	1-Phenyl-2, 4-hexadiene
0.05%	-	Dill apiole
45.55	TOTAL %	13 COMPOUNDS

Artemisia speciosa (China)

BOTANICAL SPECIES

Artemisia speciosa (Pamp.) Ling et Y.R. Ling, fam. Asteraceae (Compositae)

AUTHOR

Liangfeng Zhu, Li Yonghua, Li Baoiing, Lu Biyao & Xia Nianhe

TITLE

Aromatic Plants and Essential Constituents p. 284

PUBLICATION

South China Institute of Botany, Chinese Academy of Sciences, Hai Feng Publishing Co., Chinese National Node for APINMAP, distributed by Peace Book Co. Ltd., Hong Kong (1993)

COMPOUNDS

52.53%	-	alpha-Thujone
16.25%	-	cis-Sabinol
7.28%	-	iso-alpha-Thujone
2.56%	-	Camphor
2.04%	-	Sabinol
2.00%	-	Valeranone
1.40%	-	Artemisia ketone
1.03%	-	3-Hexenyl butyrate
0.79%	-	1, 8-Cineole
0.78%	-	alpha-Selinol
0.70%	-	Borneol
0.40%	-	Terpinen-4-ol
0.25%	-	alpha-Bisabolol
0.16%	-	2.4-He.xadienol
88.17	TOTAL %	14 COMPOUNDS

Artemisia subulata (China)

BOTANICAL SPECIES

Artemisia subulata Nakai, fam. Asteraceae (Compositae)

AUTHOR

Liangfeng Zhu, Li Yonghua, Li Baoling, Lu Biyao & Xia Nianhe

TITLE

Aromatic Plants and Essential Constituents p. 285

PUBLICATION

South China Institute of Botany, Chinese Academy of Sciences, Hai Feng Publishing Co., Chinese National Node for APINMAP, distributed by Peace Book Co. Ltd., Hong Kong (1993)

COMPOUNDS

48.97%	-	1, 8-Cineole	
19.87%	-	Camphor	
7.95%	-	Borneol	
4.20%	-	Terpinen-4-ol	
2.99%	-	alpha-Terpineol	
1.33%	-	beta-Selinene	
0.79%	-	beta-Caryophyllene	
0.76%	-	alpha-Selinol	
0.56%	-	beta-Cubebene	
0.53%	-	gamma-Terpinene	
0.53%	-	7-Octen-4-ol	
0.29%	-	2-Hexenal	
0.23%	-	Eugenol	
0.19%	-	Carveol	
0.16%	-	alpha-Terpinene	
89.35		TOTAL %	15 COMPOUNDS

Artemisia umbelliformis (Italy)

BOTANICAL SPECIES

Artemisia umbelliformis Lam., fam. Asteraceae (Compositae)

AUTHOR

Mucciarelli, M., Caramiello, R., Maffei, M., and Chialva, F.

TITLE

Essential Oils from Some Artemisia Species Growing Spontaneously in North-West Italy (0.01% = trace)

PUBLICATION

Flavour Fragr. J., Vol. 10, 25-32 (1995)

COMPOUNDS

67.50%	-	alpha-Thujone
18.20%	-	beta-Thujone
2.00%	-	1, 8-Cineole
1.60%	-	Sabinene
1.60%	-	Sabinyl acetate
1.30%	-	Terpinen-4-ol
1.00%	-	para-Cymene
0.70%	-	beta-Pinene
0.70%	-	Carvacrol
0.60%	-	gamma-Terpinene
0.60%	-	gamma-Selinene
0.50%	-	beta-Caryophyllene
0.40%	-	Camphor
0.40%	-	Caryophyllene oxide
0.40%	-	cis-2-Thujenol-4
0.30%	-	alpha-Thujene
0.30%	-	alpha-Pinene

0.30%	-	alpha-Terpinene
0.20%	-	alpha-Copaene
0.20%	-	trans-Sabinene hydrate
0.20%	-	Pinocarvone
0.20%	-	Cuminaldehyde
0.10%	-	Limonene
0.10%	-	Terpinolene
0.10%	-	Myrtenal
0.10%	-	Myrtenol
0.10%	-	Spathulenol
0.10%	-	Linalool oxides (cis/trans) (unknown isomers)
0.01%	-	Camphene
0.01%	-	Myrcene
0.01%	-	alpha-Phellandrene
0.01%	-	Linalool
0.01%	-	Borneol
0.01%	-	alpha-Terpineol
0.01%	-	Carvone
0.01%	-	Bornyl acetate
0.01%	-	trans-Pinocarveol
0.01%	-	dehydro-1, 8-Cineole
0.01%	-	Yomogi alcohol
0.01%	-	Artemisia alcohol
0.01%	-	trans-Verbenol
0.01%	-	(E)-Nerolidol
0.01%	-	alpha-Cadinol
0.01%	-	Verbenone
0.01%	-	alpha-Fenchene
0.01%	-	trans-Carveol
0.01%	-	aipha-Bisabolol

0.01%	-	Artemisia ketone
0.01%	-	cis-Chrysanthenyl acetate
0.01%	-	beta-Damascenone
0.01%	-	Ascaridole
0.01%	-	Camphenilone
0.01%	-	epi-Cubebol
0.01%	-	Isopinocamphone
0.01%	-	trans-alpha-Bergamotol
0.01%	-	trans-Chrysantenyl acetate
0.01%	-	cis-Ocimene epoxide
0.01%	-	Nojigiku alcohol
0.01%	-	Bisabolol oxide (unknown isomer)
100.11	TOTAL %	59 COMPOUNDS

Artemisia valiesiaca (Italy)

BOTANICAL SPECIES

Artemisia vallesiaca All., fam. Asteraceae (Compositae)

AUTHOR

Mucciarelli, M., Caramiello, R., Maffei, M., and Chialva, F.

TITLE

Essential Oils from Some Artemisia Species Growing Spontaneously in North-West Italy (0.01-% = trace)

PUBLICATION

Flavour Fragr. J., Vol. 10, 25-32 (1995)

COMPOUNDS

40.50%	-	Camphor
27.70%	-	Borneol
15.10%	-	1, 8-Cineole
7.40%	-	Camphene
2.80%	-	Verbenone
0.90%	-	trans-Verbenol
0.60%	-	para-Cymene
0.50%	-	Terpinen-4-ol
0.50%	-	Carvone
0.50%	-	Spathulenol
0.30%	-	Bornyl acetate
0.30%	-	Myrtenal
0.30%	-	Carveol
0.20%	-	beta-Pinene
0.20%	-	beta-Caryophyllene
0.20%	-	beta-Selinene
0.20%	-	alpha-Thujone

0.20%	-	trans-Pinocarveol
0.20%	-	Caryophyllene oxide
0.20%	-	Sabinene hydrate
0.10%	-	alpha-Pinene
0.10%	-	alpha-Terpinene
0.10%	-	Limonene
0.10%	-	gamma-Terpinene
0.10%	-	alpha-Terpineol
0.10%	-	beta-Thujone
0.10%	-	dehydro-1, 8-Cineole
0.10%	-	Pinocarvone
0.10%	-	Linalool oxides (cis/trans) (unknown isomers)
0.10%	-	cis-2-Thujenol-4
0.01%	-	alpha-Thujene
0.01%	-	Sabinene
0.01%	-	Myrcene
0.01%	-	alpha-Phellandrene
0.01%	-	Terpinolene
0.01%	-	Linalool
0.01%	-	aipha-Copaene
0.01%	-	Yomogi alcohol
0.01%	-	Artemisia alcohol
0.01%	-	Myrtenol
0.01%	-	Carvacrol
0.01%	-	(E)-Nerolidol
0.01%	-	Cubenol
0.01%	-	alpha-Cadinol
0.01%	-	alpha-Fenchene
0.01%	-	alpha-Bisabolol
0.01%	-	Cuminaldehyde

0.01%	-	Artemisia ketone
0.01%	-	Artemisyl acetate
0.01%	-	cis-Chrysanthenyl acetate
0.01%	-	beta-Damascenone
0.01%	-	Ascaridole
0.01%	-	Camphenilone
0.01%	-	Isopinocarnphone
0.01%	-	trans-afpha-Bergamotol
0.01%	-	cis-Sabinyl acetate
0.01%	-	trans-Chrysantenyl acetate
0.01%	-	cis-Ocimene epoxide
0.01%	-	Nojigiku alcohol
0.01%	-	Bisabolol oxide (unknown isomer)
100.10	TOTAL %	60 COMPOUNDS

Artemisia verlotiorum (Italy)

BOTANICAL SPECIES

Artemisia verlotiorum Lamotte, fam. Asteraceae (Compositae)

AUTHOR

Mucciarelli, M., Caramiello, R., Maffei, M., and Chialva, F.

TITLE

Essential Oils from Some Artemisia Species Growing Spòntaneously in North-West Italy (0.01%= trace)

PUBLICATION

Flavour Fragr. J., Vol. 10, 25-32 (1995)

COMPOUNDS

21.40%	-	Caryophyllene oxide
17.60%	-	Borneol
11.20%	-	Camphor
10.60%	-	1, 8-Cineole
9.20%	-	Spathulenol
7.60%	-	trans-Verbenol
3.80%	-	Myrcene
3.70%	-	alpha-Fenchene
3.40%	-	Cuminaldehyde
3.30%	-	Limonene
2.70%	-	para-Cymene
2.10%	-	Myrtenol
1.10%	-	alpha-Copaene
1.10%	-	dehydro-1, 8-Cineole
0.80%	-	alpha-Thujene
0.60%	-	alpha-Pinene

0.01% - Camphene
0.01% - Sabinene
0.01% - beta-Pinene
0.01% - alpha-Phellandrene
0.01% - alpha-Terpinene
0.01% - gamma-Terpinene
0.01% - Terpinolene
0.01% - Linalool
0.01% - Terpinen-4-ol
0.01% - alpha-Terpineol
0.01% - Carvone
0.01% - Bornyl acetate
0.01% - beta-Caryophyllene
0.01% - Myrtenal
0.01% - alpha-Thujone
0.01% - beta-Thujone
0.01% - Yomogi alcohol
0.01% - Artemisia alcohol
0.01% - Pinocarvone
0.01% - Carvacrol
0.01% - Sabinene hydrate
0.01% - (E)-Nerolidol
0.01% - alpha-Cadinol
0.01% - Pinocarveol
0.01% - Verbenone
0.01% - trans-Carveol
0.01% - alpha-Bisabolol
0.01% - Artemisia ketone
0.01% - Artemisyl acetate
0.01% - cis-Chrysanthenyl acetate
0.01% - Linalool oxides (cis/trans) (unknown

		isomers)
0.01%	-	beta-Damascenone
0.01%	-	Ascaridole
0.01%	-	gamrna-Selinene
0.01%	-	1-epi-Cubenol
0.01%	-	Camphenilone
0.01%	-	Isopinocamphone
0.01%	-	trans-alpha-Bergamotol
0.01%	-	Sabinyl acetate
0.01%	-	trans-Chrysantenyl acetate
0.01%	-	cis-Ocimene epoxide
0.01%	-	cis-2-Thujenol-4
0.01%	-	Nojigiku alcohol
0.01%	-	Bisabolol oxide (unknown isomer)
100.64		TOTAL % 60 COMPOUNDS

Artemisia vestita (India)

BOTANICAL SPECIES

Artemisia vestita Wall. ex Dc., fam. Asteraceae (Compositae)

AUTHOR

Thakur, R.S., and Misra, L.N.

TITLE

Essential Oils of Indian Artemisia

PUBLICATION

In: Proceedings 11th Intern. Congress of Essential Oils, Fragrances and Flavours, 12-16 Dec., 1989, New Delhi, India, Vol. 4, 127-135

COMPOUNDS

10.10%	-	beta-Himachalene
6.85%	-	alpha-Atlantone
5.30%	-	1, 8-Cineole
5.00%	-	Himachalol
4.50%	-	Artemisia alcohol
3.14%	-	Santolina alconol
3.00%	-	Artemisyl acetate
2.90%	-	Himachalol (isomer)
2.82%	-	gamma-Himachalene
2.82%	-	alpha-Himachalene
2.63%	-	Yomogi alcohol
2.35%	-	beta-Caryophllene
1.82%	-	alpha-Thujone
1.56%	-	Germacrene D
1.19%	-	cis-Chrysanthenyl acetate
1.13%	-	Camphor

1.06%	-	Sabinene hydrate
0.90%	-	alpha-Phellandrene
0.85%	-	Borneol
0.83%	-	Sabinol
0.78%	-	para-Cymene
0.78%	-	Artemisia ketone
0.69%	-	beta-Thujone
0.56%	-	alpha-Pinene
0.53%	-	cis-p-Menth-2-en-l-ol
0.52%	-	Camphene
0.51%	-	Fragranol
0.46%	-	Sabinene
0.45%	-	trans-Piperitol
0.41%	-	Terpinen-4-ol
0.38%	-	cis-Chrysanthenol
0.35%	-	Santolinatriene
0.35%	-	beta-Pinene
0.35%	-	cis-Sabinene hydrate
0.35%	-	Chrysanthenone
0.27%	-	Myrcene
0.23%	-	Limonene
0.21%	-	alpha-Terpineol
0.20%	-	Linalool
0.15%	-	cis-Piperitol
69.27	TOTAL %	40 COMPOUNDS

Armoise flower

BOTANICAL SPECIES

Artemisia vulgaris L., fam. Asteraceae (Compositae)

AUTHOR

Michaelis, K. et al.

TITLE

Das aetherische Oel aus Blueten von Artemisia vulgaris L.

PUBLICATION

Z. Naturforsch. Vol. 37 C, 152-158 (1982)

COMPOUNDS

15.88%	-	Sabinene
13.67%	-	Myrcene
9.75%	-	1, 8-Cineole
6.00%	-	beta-Cubebene
3.41%	-	delta-Guaiene
2.17%	-	Vulgarol
1.93%	-	Terpinen-4-ol
1.84%	-	Camphor
1.64%	-	gamma-Terpinene
1.53%	-	gamma-Elemene
1.44%	-	Camphene
1.43%	-	beta-Pinene
1.42%	-	alpha-Thujene
1.29%	-	alpha-Pinene
1.13%	-	trans-Sabinene hydrate
0.91%	-	para-Cymene
0.83%	-	alpha-Terpinene
0.71%	-	(E)-beta-Ocimene

0.71%	-	Borneol
0.67%	-	beta-Caryophyllene
0.46%	-	Terpinolene
0.36%	-	delta-Cadinene
0.30%	-	Methyl eugenol
0.28%	-	alpha-Terpineol
0.21%	-	gamma-Cadinene
0.20%	-	Decanal
0.17%	-	Isoborneol
0.15%	-	alpha-Humulene
0.12%	-	Perillaldehyde
0.12%	-	beta-Elemene
0.12%	-	Aromadendrene
0.11%	-	alpha-Terpinyl acetate
0.10%	-	Bomyl acetate
0.10%	-	cis-Piperitol
0.09%	-	Myrtenol
0.08%	-	alpha-Phellandrene
0.08%	-	cis-Sabinene hydrate
0.06%	-	Cuminaldehyde
0.06%	-	Nonanal
0.06%	-	Geranial
0.06%	-	Perillene
0.05%	-	Undecanal
0.05%	-	alpha-Copaene
0.05%	-	alpha-Cubebene
0.05%	-	Nonadien-3-one (unknown structure)
0.05%	-	Tolualdehyde (unknown structure)
0.05%	-	allo-Aromadendrene
0.04%	-	Limonene
0.04%	-	(Z)-beta-Ocimene

0.03%	-	Carvone	
0.03%	-	Isopiperitenone	
0.02%	-	Carvacrol	
0.01%	-	Neryl acetate	
0.01%	-	Geranyl acetate	
0.01%	-	Methyl chavicol	
72.15		TOTAL %	55 COMPOUNDS

Artemisia vulgaris (Italy)

BOTANICAL SPECIES

Artemisia vulgaris L., Cam. Asteraceae (Compositae)

AUTHOR

Mucciarelli, M., Caramiello, R., Maffei, M., and Chialva, F.

TITLE

Essential Oils from Some Artemisia Species Growing Spontaneously in North-West Italy (0.01% = trace)

PUBLICATION

Flavour Fragr. J., Vol. 10, 25-32

COMPOUNDS

47.70%	-	Camphor
9.10%	-	Camphene
8.60%	-	Verbenone
7.00%	-	trans-Verbenol
4.30%	-	beta-Caryophyllene
3.90%	-	1, 8-Cineole
2.40%	-	gamma-Selinene
2.20%	-	Caryophyllene oxide
2.10%	-	alpha-Thujene
2.10%	-	beta-Pinene
2.00%	-	alpha-Pinene
1-30%	-	Spathulenol
1.10%	-	alpha-Copaene
0.90%	-	Limonene
0.70%	-	Bornyl acetate
0.70%	-	Myrtenol
0.60%	-	para-Cymene

0.40%	-	Borneol
0.40%	-	Terpinen-4-ol
0.30%	-	gamma-Terpinene
0.30%	-	alpha-Terpineol
0.30%	-	Nojigiku alcohol
0.30%	-	Bisabolol oxide (unknown isomer)
0.20%	-	Carvacrol
0.20%	-	Pinocarveol
0.20%	-	cis-Chrysanthenyl acetate
0 10%	-	Myrcene
0.10%	-	alpha-Terpinene
0.10%	-	Terpinolene
0.10%	-	Linalool
0.10%	-	Ascaridole
0.10%	-	Sabinyl acetate
0.01%	-	Sabinene
0.01%	-	alpha-Phellandrene
0.01%	-	Carvone
0.01%	-	alpha-Thujone
0.01%	-	beta-Thujone
0.01%	-	Myrtenal
0.01%	-	dehydro-1, 8-Cineole
0.01%	-	Yomogi alcohol
0.01%	-	Artemisia alcohol
0.01%	-	Pinocarvone
0.01%	-	Sabinene hydrate
0.01%	-	(E)-Nerolidol
0.01%	-	alpha-Cadinol
0.01%	-	alpha-Fenchene
0.01%	-	trans-Carveol
0.01%	-	alpha-Bisabolol

0.01%	-	Cuminaldehyde
0.01%	-	Artemisia kétone
0.01%	-	Artemisyl acetate
0.01%	-	Linalool oxides (cis/trans) (unknown isomers)
0.01%	-	beta-Damascenone
0.01%	-	1-epi-Cubenol
0.01%	-	Camphenilone
0.01%	-	Isopinocamphone
0.01%	-	trans-alpha-Bergamotol
0.01%	-	trans-Chrysaritenyl acetate
0.01%	-	cis-Ocimene epoxide
0.01%	-	cis-2-Thujenol-4
100.18	TOTAL %	60 COMPOUNDS

Artemisia Waltonii (China)

BOTANICAL SPECIES

Artemisia waltonii J.R. Drumm. ex Pamp., fam. Asteraceae (Compositae)

AUTHOR

Liangfeng Zhu, Li Yonghua, Li Baoling, Lu Biyao & Xia Nianhe

TITLE

Aromatic Plants and Essential Constituents p. 286

PUBLICATION

South China Institute of Botany, Chinese Academy of Sciences, Hai Feng Publishing Co., Chinese National Node for APINNAP, distributed by Peace Book Co. Ltd., Hong Kong (1993)

COMPOUNDS

33.64%	-	Elemicin
32.06%	-	Methyl eugenol
5.48%	-	Cumin alcohol
1.42%	-	2, 6-di-tert-Butyl-p-cresol
1.03%	-	1, 8-Cineole
0.87%	-	(2-Hydroxy-5-methylphenyl)-ethanone
0.80%	-	Capillene
0.79%	-	Bornyl acetate
0.58%	-	m-Anisaldehyde
0.35%	-	Capillinone
0.34%	-	Borneol
0.33%	-	alpha-Terpineol
0.30%	-	Linalool
0.22%	-	alpha-Curcumene
0.21	-	Farnesol (unknown isomer)
78.42	TOTAL %	15 COMPOUNDS

Baccharis genistelloides

BOTANICAL SPECIES

Baccharis genistelloides Pers. (Carqueja), fam. Asteraceae (Compositae)

AUTHOR

Chialva, F., and Doglia, G.

TITLE

Essential oil from Carqueja (Baccharis genistelloides Pers.)

PUBLICATION

J. Ess. Oil Res., Vol, 173-177 (July/August 1990)

COMPOUNDS

42.82%	-	Carquejyl acetate
8.24%	-	beta-Pinene
5.74%	-	Calacorene (unknown isomer)
4.34%	-	Germacrene D
3.49%	-	beta-Elemene
3.47%	-	(E)-beta-Ocimene
2.65%	-	Limonene
2.03%	-	beta-Phellandrene
2.03%	-	Carquejol
1.58%	-	Bicyclogermacrene
1.43%	-	beta-Eudesmol
1.41%	-	alpha-Ylangene
1.34%	-	beta-Caryophyllene
1.29%	-	Sabinene
1.26%	-	Sesquiterpene hydrocarbons (unknown)
1.04%	-	Ledol
0.84%	-	Viridiflorol

0.75%	-	Myrcene
0.68%	-	(Z)-beta-Famesene
0.63%	-	Cyperene
0.52%	-	alpha-Muurolene
0.51%	-	3, 6, 6-Trimethyl-2,4-cycloheptadien-1-one
0.44%	-	Ledene
0.39%	-	Elemol
0.29%	-	Spathutenol
0.28%	-	Chrysanthenone
0.28%	-	Monoterpenyl esters
0.24%	-	beta-Cubebene
0.20%	-	alpha-Pinene
0.20%	-	delta-Cadinene
0.18%	-	alpha-Cubebene
0.18%	-	alpha, p-Dimethylstyrene
0.16%	-	Terpinolene
0.10%	-	Camphene
0.10%	-	gamma-Terpinene
0.09%	-	(Z)-beta-Ocimene
0.09%	-	2-Methyl-6-methylene-1,7-octadien-3-one
0.08%	-	Palustrol
0.08%	-	(Z)-Methyl isoeugeol
0.07%	-	Linalool
0.07%	-	delta-Elemene
0.06%	-	alpha-phellandrene
0.06%	-	para-Cymene
0.05%	-	alpha-Terpinene
0.01%	-	1, 8-Cineole
0.01%	-	alpha-Copaene
0.01%	-	Eudesmols (unknown isomer)
91.81	TOTAL%	47 COMPOUNDS

Blumea brevipes

BOTANICAL SPECIES

Blumea brevipes (Oliv. & Hiern) Willd., fam. Asteraceae (Compositae)

AUTHOR

Mwangi, J.W., K.J. Achola, W. Lwande, A. Hassanali & R. Laurent

TITLE

Constituents of the Essential Oil of Biumea brevipes (Oliv. & Hiern) Willd.

PUBLICATION

Flavour Fragr. J., Vol. 9, 233-235 (1994)

COMPOUNDS

27.60% - Terpinen-4-ol
15.40% - Germacrene D
8.00% - Sabinene
5.50% - gamma-Terpinene
4.00% - delta-Cadinene
3.90% - (E)-beta-Ocimene
3.10% - trans-Sabinene hydrate
2.60% - alpha-Terpinene
2.40% - beta-Bourbonene
1.90% - alpha-Pinene
1.90% - Terpinolene
1.90% - alpha-Cadinol
1.50% - alpha-Terpineol
1.50% - Elemol
1.20% - Linalool
1.00% - alpha-Thujene

0.90%	-	l-Octenol-3
0.80%	-	Myrcene
0.80%	-	alpha-Copaene
0.70%	-	beta-Selinene
0.60%	-	para-Cymene
0.60%	-	alpha-Humulene
0.50%	-	beta-Phellandrene
0.40%	-	cis-Sabinene hydrate
0.40%	-	T-Muurolol
0.40%	-	trans-p-Menth-2-en-l-ol
0.40%	-	cis-3-Hexenyl 2-methylbutyrate
0.30%	-	Camphene
0.30%	-	Limonene
0.30%	-	Camphor
0.30%	-	beta-Cubebene
0.30%	-	beta-Eudesmol
0.30%	-	alpha-Eudesmol
0.20%	-	Caryophyllene oxide
0.20%	-	cis-p-Menth-2-en-l-ol
0.20%	-	Thymohydroquinone dimethylether
0.20%	-	Benzyl 2-methylbutyrate
0.10%	-	beta-Pinene
0.10%	-	(Z)-beta-Ocimene
0.10%	-	Sesquiterpene alcohols (unknown)
0.10%	-	1-Hexanol
0.05%	-	Geranyl acetate
0.05%	-	beta-Caryophyllene
0.05%	-	alpha-Muurolene
0.05%	-	beta-Thujone
0.05%	-	cis-Piperitol
0.05%	-	trans-Piperitol
0.05%	-	Spathulenol

0.05%	-	beta-Elemene
0.05%	-	(E)-Nerolidol
0.05%	-	Cubenol
0.05%	-	alpha-Selinene
0.05%	-	allo-Aromadendrene
0.05%	-	(Z)-3-Hexenol
0.05%	-	3-Octanol
0.05%	-	alpha-Cadinene
0.05%	-	Humulene oxide
0.05%	-	alpha-Calacorene
0.05%	-	Methyl salicylate
0.05%	-	1-epi-Cubenol
0.05%	-	(Z)-3-Hexenyl acetate
0.05%	-	Torreyol
0.05%	-	(-)-Germacra-1, 6-dien-5-ol
0.05%	-	3-Octanone
0.05%	-	trans-Calamenene
0.05%	-	4, 8-Dimethylnona-1,3,7-triene
0.02%	-	beta-Bisabolene
0.02%	-	Bicyclogermacrene
95.19		TOTAL % 69 COMPOUNDS

Blumea lanceolaria

BOTANICAL SPECIES

Blumea lanceolaria (Roxb.) Druce, fam. Asteraceae (Compositae)

AUTHOR

Nguyêñ Xuân Duñg, Dô Tat Loi, Dô Tât hung and Leclercq P.A.

TITLE

Chemical composition of the Oil of Blumea lanceolaria (Roxb.) Druce from Vietnam

PUBLICATION

J. Ess. Oil Res., Vol.3, 285-286 (Jul/Aug 1991)

COMPOUNDS

94.96%	-	Methyl thymol	
3.28%	-	para-Cymene	
0.79%	-	1-Hexadecanol	
0.12%	-	Limonene	
0.04%	-	alpha-Thujene	
0.04%	-	beta-Caryophyllene	
0.02%	-	Methyl carvacrol	
0.01%	-	alpha-Pinene	
0.01%	-	Camphene	
0.01%	-	beta-Pinene	
0.01%	-	alpha-Terpinene	
99.29		TOTAL %	11 COMPOUNDS

Muhuhu

BOTANICAL SPECIES

Brachylaena hutchinsii Hutch. (Synchodendron hutchii Hutch.), Asteraceae

AUTHOR

Klein, E., and Schmidt, W.

TITLE

The main constituents of Muhuhu oil

PUBLICATION

Dragoco Rept., (5), 87-91 (1973).

COMPOUNDS

16.50%	-	alpha-Amorphene
10.00%	-	Brachyl oxide
7.50%	-	Copaenal
7.50%	-	Copaenol
6.50%	-	delta-Cadinene
5.00%	-	Sesquiterpene alcohols (unknown)
5.00%	-	alpha-Calacorene
4.50%	-	Cyclic ether (unknown structure)
4.00%	-	Ylangenal
3.50%	-	Cubebol
3.00%	-	alpha-Muurolene
3.00%	-	Cadalene
2.00%	-	alpha-Copaene
1.50%	-	Ylangenol
1.00%	-	alpha-Ylangene
1.00%	-	gamma-Amorphene
0.50%	-	Calamenene
82.00	TOTAL %	17 COMPOUNDS

Marigold pot 1

BOTANICAL SPECIES

Calendula officinalis L. (Pot Marigold), fam. Asteraceae (Compositae)

AUTHOR

Chalchat, J.C., Carry, R.Ph., and Michet, A.

TITLE

Chemical Composition of Essential Oil of Calendula officinalis L. (Pot Marigold) (oil of complete plant: relative percentages)

PUBLICATION

Flav. Fragr. J, Vol. 6, 189-192 (1991)

COMPOUNDS

25.13%	-	alpha-Cadinol
14.86%	-	delta-Cadinene
7.46%	-	beta-Fenchene
7.04%	-	10-alpha-Muurolol
5.16%	-	T-Cadinol
2.75%	-	Nerolidol (unknown isomer)
2.10%	-	alpha-Pinene
1.87%	-	T-Muurolol
1.60%	-	Cadinene (unknown isomer)
1.30%	-	alpha-Patchoulene
1.11%	-	beta-Cubebene
1.11%	-	Cubenene (unknown structure)
1.08%	-	alpha-Cadinene
1.00%	-	gamma-Muurolene
0.98%	-	Terpinen-4-ol
0.98%	-	epi-Cubebol

0.80% - Cubebol
0.77% - alpha-Humulene
0.63% - beta-Ylangene
0.62% - gamma-Terpinene
0.60% - Sabinene
0.53% - Limonene
0.52% - Myrcene
0.44% - Eudesmols (unknown isomer)
0.42% - beta-Phellandrene
0.38% - Cubebene (unknown isomer)
0.37% - beta-Caryophyllene
0.33% - alpha-Muurolene
0 28% - beta-Pinene
0.27% - para-Cymene
0.26% - Aromadendrene
0.24% - Calacorene (unknown isomer)
0.23% - (E)-beta-Ocimene
0.22% - alpha-Terpinene
0.22% - Bornyl acetate
0.19% - 1, 8-Cineole
0.17% - Camphene
0.17% - alpha-Cubebene
0.16% - gamma-Amorphene
0.14% - alpha-Phellandrene
0.14% - gamma-Cadinene
0.14% - Calamenene
0.11% - Terpinolene
0.10% - delta-3-Carene
0.10% - alpha-Gurjunene
0.09% - Menthone
0.05% - gamma-Patchoutene

0.07%	-	beta-Farnesene	
0.05%	-	Camphor	
0.04%	-	alpha-Copaene	
0.03%	-	(Z)-beta-Ocimene	
0.01%	-	2-Butanone	
0.01%	-	2-Pentanone	
85.46		TOTAL %	53 COMPOUNDS

Marigold pot 2

BOTANICAL SPECIES

Calendula officinalis L. (Pot Marigold), fam. Asteraceae (Compositae)

AUTHOR

Chalchat, J.C., Carry, R.Ph., and Michet, A.

TITLE

Chemical Composition of Essential Oil of Calendula officinalis L. (Pot Marigold) (flower oils: relative percentages)

PUBLICATION

Flav. Fragr. J., Vol. 6, 1891-92 (1991)

COMPOUNDS

20.09%	-	alpha-Cadinol
8.14%	-	Nerolidol (unknown isomer)
7.83%	-	Eudesmols (unknown isomer)
7.26%	-	10-epi-Cubenol
5.67%	-	10-alpha-Muurolol
5.30%	-	delta-Cadinene
3.21%	-	T-Cadinol
2.93%	-	alpha-Patchoulene
2.53%	-	beta-Cubebene
2.25%	-	Aromadendrene
1.37%	-	Bornyl acetate
1.17%	-	Limonene
1.06%	-	T-Muurolol
0.94%	-	alpha-Humulene
0.82%	-	cis-Caryophyllene
0.70%	-	Cadinene (unknown isomer)

0.65%	-	beta-Fenchene
0.59%	-	para-Cymene
0.59%	-	Cubenol
0.58%	-	alpha-Gurjunene
0.46%	-	alpha-Cadinene
0.45%	-	gamma-Muurolene
0.40%	-	(E)-beta-Ocimene
0.37%	-	gamma-Terpinene
0.31%	-	gamma-Cadinene
0.25%	-	beta-Phellandrene
0.24%	-	beta-Pinene
0.22%	-	beta-Farnesene
0.21%	-	delta-3-Carene
0.20%	-	alpha-Pinene
0.20%	-	2-Butanone
0.17%	-	Myrcene
0.17%	-	Cubebene (unknown isomer)
0.13%	-	beta-Ylangene
0.12%	-	alpha-Terpinene
0.11%	-	Sabinene
0.11%	-	alpha-Cubebene
0.10%	-	Calamenene
0.10%	-	gamma-Amorphene
0.09%	-	Terpinolene
0.05%	-	Menthone
0.04%	-	Terpinen-4-ol
0.04%	-	2-Pentanone
0.02%	-	Camphene
0.02%	-	alpha-Phellandrene
78.26		TOTAL % 45 COMPOUNDS

Chamomile (Argentina)

BOTANICAL SPECIES

Chamomilla recutita (L.) Rausch. (Matricaria chamomilla L.), fam.Asteraceae

AUTHOR

Malinskas, G.A.G., Santi, M.N., and Retamar, J.A.

TITLE

Aceite Esencial de Matricaria chamomilla L. (Manzanilla)

PUBLICATION

Essenze Deriv. Agrum., Vol. 55 (1), 52 61 (1985)

COMPOUNDS

46.11%	-	alpha-Bisabolol oxide A
15.42%	-	Famesene (unknown isomer)
3.32%	-	1, 4, 9, 9-Tetramethyloctahydro-1H,3a,7 methylazulene (tent.)
1.93%	-	Farnesol (unknown isomer)
1.93%	-	Nerolidol (unknown isomer)
1.22%	-	1, 5-Dimethyl-6-methylenespiro [2,4]heptane (tent.)
1.06%	-	beta-Caryophyllene
1.05%	-	Chamazulene
1.01%	-	Pulegone
0.57%	-	1, 8-Cineole
0.31%	-	alpha-Terpineol
0.26%	-	Myrcene
0.20%	-	Borneol
0.08%	-	Linalool
74.47	TOTAL %	14 COMPOUNDS

Chamomile (Hungary)

BOTANICAL SPECIES

Chamomilla recutita (L.) Rausch. (Matricaria chamomilla L.), fam.Asteraceae

AUTHOR

Schilcher, H.

TITLE

Neuere Erkenntnisse bei der Qualitaetsbeurteilung von Kamillenblueten bzw. Kamillenoel

PUBLICATION

Deut. Apoth. Ztg., Vol. 112, 1497-1500 (1972); Planta Med., Vol. 23, 132-144 (1973)

COMPOUNDS

20.00%	-	alpha-Bisabolol oxide B
20.00%	-	alpha-Bisabolol oxide A
10.00%	-	alpha-Bisabolol
8.00%	-	Chamazulene
7.00%	-	Spiro ether
65.00	TOTAL %	5 COMPOUNDS

Chamomile (Brazil)

BOTANICAL SPECIES

Chamomilla recutita (L.) Rausch. (Matricaria chamomilla L.), fam. Asteraceae

AUTHOR

Matos, F.J.A., M.I.L. Machado, J.W. Alencar & A.A. Craveiro

TITLE

Constituents of Brazilian Chamomile Oil

PUBLICATION

J. Essent. Oil Res., Vol. 5, 337-339 (May/Jun 1993)

COMPOUNDS

23.54%	-	alpha-Bisabolol oxide B
16.85%	-	alpha-Bisabolol oxide A
15.97%	-	(Z)-beta-Farnesene
13.15%	-	alpha-Bisabolol
8.19%	-	Chamazulene
5.21%	-	alpha-Bisabolone oxide
4.71%	-	Chamospiroether
0.75%	-	gamma-Cadinene
88.37	TOTAL %	8 COMPOUNDS

Chamomile (Germany) 1

BOTANICAL SPECIES

Chamomilla recutita (L.) Rausch. (Matricaria chamomilla L), fam. Asteraceae

AUTHOR

Brunke, E.-J., F.-J. Hammerschmidt & G. Schmaus

TITLE

Die Headspace-Analyse von Bluetendueften (analysis of steamdistilled oil)

PUBLICATION

Dragoco Report 1/1992, 3-31

COMPOUNDS

57.68%	-	alpha-Bisabolol oxide A
23.35%	-	Chamazulene
4.35%	-	alpha-Bisabolol oxide B
4.10%	-	alpha-Bisabolone oxide
2.92%	-	(E)-beta-Farnesene
1.48%	-	Germacrene D
0.70%	-	(E)-beta-Ocimene
0.64%	-	Bicyclogermacrene
0 51%	-	alpha-Bisabolol
0.51%	-	Artemisia ketone
0.39%	-	Artemisia alcohol
0.34%	-	1, 8-Cineole
0-22%	-	Sabinene
0.17%	-	Ethyl 2-methylbutyrate
0.10%	-	(E)-2-Hexenol
0.09%	-	beta-Caryophyllene

0.08%	-	(Z)-beta-Ocimene
0.07%	-	para-Cymene
001%	-	alpha-Pinene
0.01%	-	Myrcene
0.01%	-	Limonene
0.01%	-	Terpinen-4-ol
0.01%	-	beta-Selinene
0.01%	-	6-Methyl-5-hepten-2-one
0.01%	-	(2)-3-Hexenyl acetate
0.01%	-	Propyl 2-methylbutyrate
97.78		TOTAL % 26 COMPOUNDS

Chainomile (Germany) 2, Living Flower

BOTANICAL SPECIES

Chamomilla recutita (L.) Rausch. (Matricaria chamomilla L.), fam. Asteraceae

AUTHOR

Brunke, E.-J., F.-J. Hammerschmidt & G. Schmaus

TITLE

Die Headspace-Aanalyse von Bluetendueften (analysis by closed loop stripping of living flowers)

PUBLICATION

Dragoco Report 1/1992, 3-31

COMPOUNDS

22.23%	-	para-Cymene
15.97%	-	beta-Selinene
10.34%	-	Artemisia ketone
8.75%	-	1, 8-Cineole
6.95%	-	(Z)-3-Hexenyl acetate
6.15%	-	Ethyl 2-methylbutyrate
5.10%	-	beta-Caryopnyllene
4.90%	-	(E)-beta-Farnesene
2 22%	-	Propyl 2-methylbutyrate
1.26%	-	alpha-Pinene
1.15%	-	alpha-Bisabolone oxide
0.97%	-	Limonene
0.92%	-	Bicyclogermacrene
0.75%	-	Myrcene
0.51%	-	Artemisia alcohol
0.45%	-	(E)-2-Hexenol

0.39%	-	Sabinene
0.37%	-	(Z)-3-Hexenyl propionate
0.37%	-	2, 6-Dimethyl-3(E),5(E),7-octatrien-2-ol
0.33%	-	alpha-Humulene
0.32%	-	Lavandulyl acetate
0.31%	-	(Z)-3-Hexenol
0.28%	-	alpha-Terpineol
0.24%	-	beta-Elemene
0.24%	-	6-Methyl-5-hepten-2-one
0.24%	-	2, 6-Dimethyl-3(E), 5(Z), 7-octatrien-2-ol
0.23%	-	Hexyl acetate
0.19%	-	alpha-Bisabolol oxide B
0.18%	-	Butyl 3-methylbutyrate
0.17%	-	alpha-Bisabolol oxide A
0.17%	-	Hexyl propionate
0.14%	-	beta-Pinene
0.14%	-	Methyl benzoate
0.12%	-	Ethyl isovalerate
0.12%	-	2, 6-Dimethyl-1,3(E),5(Z),7-octatetraene
0.12%	-	2, 6-Dimethyl-1,3(E),5(E),7-octatetraene
0.12%	-	Methyl tiglate
0.01%	-	Benzaldehyde
0.01%	-	Lavandulol
93.43	TOTAL %	39 COMPOUNDS

Carlina acaulis root

BOTANICAL SPECIES

Carlina acaulis L., fam. Asteraceae (Compositae)

AUTHOR

Chalchat, J.C., Djordjevic; S., and Gorunovic, M.

TITLE

Composition of the Essential Oil from the Root of Carlina aucalis L. Asteraceae

PUBLICATION

J. Essent. Oil Res., Vol. 8, 577-578 (Sep/Oct 1996)

COMPOUNDS

97.20%	-	Benzyl 2-furylacetylene
0.60%	-	Benzaldehyde
0.60%	-	ar-Curcumene
0.50%	-	Heptane
0.20%	-	(Z, E)-alpha-Farnesene
0.20%	-	beta-Sesquiphellandrene
0.20%	-	Phenylpropanone-2
0.05%	-	1, 8-Cineole
99.75	TOTAL %	8 COMPOUNDS

Chamomile (Bulgaria)

BOTANICAL SPECIES

Chamomilla recutita (L.) Rausch., (Matricaria chamomilla L.), fam. Asteraceae

AUTHOR

Tsutsulova A.L., and Antonova R.A.

TITLE

Analysis of Bulgarian Daisy Oil

PUBLICATION

Masio-Zhir. Prom. St., Vol. 11, 23-24 (1984)

COMPOUNDS

27.72%	-	Farnesene (unknown isomer)
17.64%	-	Chamazulene
11.17%	-	alpha-Bisabolol oxide B
9.55%	-	alpha-Bisabolol
8.93%	-	alpha-Bisabolol oxide A
5.20%	-	delta-Cadinene
3.41%	-	alpha-Muurolene
1.73%	-	(E)-beta-Ocimene
1.31%	-	gamma-Muurolene
0.50%	-	beta-Caryophyllene
0.24%	-	alpha-Copaene
0.10%	-	Limonene
0.10%	-	1, 8-Cineole
0.05%	-	para-Cymene
0.01%	-	alpha-Terpinene
87.66	TOTAL %	15 COMPOUNDS

Chamomile (Egypt)

BOTANICAL SPECIES

Chamomilla recutita (L.) Rausch.,(Matricaria chamomilla L.),fam. Asteraceae

AUTHOR

Shaath, N.A., and Azzo, N.R.

TITLE

Essential Oils of Egypt

PUBLICATION

in: Food, Flavors, Ingredients and Composition. Edit. G. Charalambous, pp. 591-603, Elsevier Sci. Publ. B.V., Amsterdam (1993)

COMPOUNDS

38.65%	-	alpha-Bisabolol oxide A
25.68%	-	(E)-beta-Farnesene
5.00%	-	alpha-Bisabolol
4.44%	-	alpha-Bisabolol oxide B
3.43%	-	Chamazulene
1.63%	-	Germacrene D
1.55%	-	alpha-Bisabolone oxide
1.30%	-	Decanoic acid
0.46%	-	Methallyl angelate
0.45%	-	delta-Cadinene
0.32%	-	(Z)-beta-Farnesene
0.21%	-	gamma-Cadinene
0.20%	-	gamma-Terpinene
0.15%	-	Ethyl 2-methylbutyrate
0.13%	-	para-Cymene
0.11%	-	Nonanal
0.08%	-	Propyl 2-methylbutyrate
83.79	TOTAL %	17 COMPOUNDS

Chamomile (Italy) 1

BOTANICAL SPECIES

Chamomilla recutita (L.) Rausch.,(Matricaria chamomilla L.), fam. Asteraceae

AUTHOR

Piccaglia R., and Marotti, M.

TITLE

Characterization of several aromatic plants grown in northern Italy (average analysis of oils of 7 cultivars grown in Ozzano (Bologna-Italy)

PUBLICATION

Flavour Fragr. J., Vol. 8, 115-122 (1993)

COMPOUNDS

40.00%	-	alpha-Bisabolol oxide A
20.00%	-	alpha-Bisabolol oxide B
10.00%	-	Chamazulene
8.00%	-	alpha-Bisabolol oxide
7.00%	-	(E)-beta-Farnesene
6.00%	-	Spiro ether
5.00%	-	alpha-Bisabolol
96.00	TOTAL %	7 COMPOUNDS

Chamomile (Italy) 2

BOTANICAL SPECIES

Chamomilla recutita (L.) Rausch.,(Matricaria chamomilla L.), fam. Asteraceae

AUTHOR

Reverchon, E., and Senatore, F.

TITLE

Supercritical carbon dioxide extraction of chamomile essential oil and its analysis by gas chromatography-mass spectrometry

PUBLICATION

J. Agric. Food Chem., Vol. 42, 154-155 (1994)

COMPOUNDS

50.42%	-	alpha-Bisabolol oxide A
16.88%	-	alpha-Bisabolol oxide B
10.00%	-	Chamospiroether
7.76%	-	alpha-Bisabolone oxide
3.52%	-	Chamazulene
1.53%	-	beta-Farnesene
0.65%	-	Nerol
0.65%	-	Spathutenol
0.57%	-	Linalool
0.42%	-	(E)-Nerolidol
0.42%	-	(Z, E)-Famesol
0.36%	-	T-Cadinol
0.35%	-	alpha-Bisabolol
0.32%	-	(E, E)-Farnesol
0.24%	-	Geraniol
0.17%	-	Caryophyllene oxide

0.17%	-	Menthyl acetate	
0.13%	-	beta-Caryophyllene	
0.11%	-	beta-Ocimene	
0.10%	-	Isoborneol	
0.09%	-	alpha-Terpineol	
0.07%	-	Terpinen-4-ol	
0.07%	-	6-Methyl-5-hepten-2-one	
0.01%	-	beta-Elemene	
0.01%	-	Menthol	
95.02		TOTAL %	25 COMPOUNDS

Chamomile, wild (Morocco)

BOTANICAL SPECIES

Ormenis mixta, fam. Asteraceae (Compositae)

AUTHOR

Toulemonde, B.

TITLE

Contribution a l'etude d'une camomille sauvage du Maroc: L'huile essentielle de I'Ormenis mixta

PUBLICATION

Parfums, Cosmet., Aromes no. 50, 65-67 (1984)

COMPOUNDS

15.00%	-	alpha-Pinene
5.00%	-	Germacrene (unknown isomer)
3.20%	-	Santolina alcohol
3 00%	-	trans-Pinocarveol
2.50%	-	Bisabolene (unknown isomer)
2,40%	-	Yomogi aicohol
2.30%	-	Artemisia alcohol
2 20%	-	Bornyl acetate
1.50%	-	beta-Caryophyllene
1.30%	-	Bornyl butyrate
1.00%	-	Myrcene
1.00%	-	Borneol
0 80%	-	Limonene
0.80%	-	delta-Cadinene
0.80%	-	Caryophyllene oxide
0.70%	-	Caryophylladienols
070%	-	delta-Elemene

0.50%	-	1, 8-Cineole
0.50%	-	Pinocarvone
0.50%	-	Cadinol (unknown structure)
0 40%	-	Camphene
0.40%	-	Santolinatriene
0.30%	-	Linalool
0.30%	-	beta-Selinene
0.30%	-	alpha-Cubebene
0 30%	-	Nerolidol (unknown isomer)
0.30%	-	Isobornyl propionate
0.25%	-	Terpinolene
0.20%	-	Sabinene
0.20%	-	Hexyl tiglate
0.10%	-	gamma-Terpinene
0.10%	-	1-Octenol-3
0.04%	-	Tricyclene
48.89	TOTAL %	33 COMPOUNDS

Balsamite

BOTANICAL SPECIES

Chrysanthemum balsamita L, fam. Asteraceae (Compositae)

AUTHOR

Bestmann, H.J., et al.

TITLE

Das aetherische Oei aus Blaettern de Balsamkrautes, C. balsamita L.

PUBLICATION

Z. Naturforsch. Vol 39c, 543-547, (1984)

COMPOUNDS

51.51%	-	Carvone
4.72%	-	beta-Cubebene
2.57%	-	Limonene
0.78%	-	alpha-Thujone
0.63%	-	1, 8-Cineole
0.50%	-	Dodecane
0.49%	-	Zingiberene
0.46%	-	Bornyl acetate
0.43%	-	Perillaldehyde
0.39%	-	(E)-beta-Farnesene
0.36%	-	cis-Carveol
0.30%	-	Pentadecane
0.24%	-	Sabinene
0.19%	-	beta-Thujone
0.15%	-	alpha-Copaene
0.12%	-	Undecane
0.11%	-	para-Cymene

0.05%	-	Terpinolene	
0.04%	-	alpha-Pinene	
0.02%	-	alpha-Fenchene	
0.01%	-	Camphene	
0.01%	-	delta-3-Carene	
64.08		TOTAL %	22 COMPOUNDS

Conyza pinnata (Zimbabwe)

BOTANICAL SPECIES

Conyza pinnata (Kuntz), fam. Asteraceae (Compositae)

AUTHOR

Petri, G., et al.

TITLE

Composition of Essential Oil from Conyza pinnata

PUBLICATION

J. Essent. Oil Res, Vol. 4, 77-78 (1992)

COMPOUNDS

39.60%	-	(E)-beta-Ocimene	
23.20%	-	Cumin alcohol	
6.95%	-	alpha-Pinene	
4.48%	-	Terpinolene	
3.91%	-	Myrcene	
2.82%	-	4-Methylacetophenone	
2.11%	-	Limonene	
1.92%	-	(Z)-beta-Ocimene	
1.05%	-	beta-Pinene	
0.85%	-	beta-Elemene	
86.89		TOTAL %	10 COMPOUNDS

Conyza sumatrensis

BOTANICAL SPECIES

Conyza sumatrensis (Retz) Walk, fam. Asteraceae (Compositaceae)

AUTHOR

Machado, S.M.F., et al.

TITLE

Essential Oil of Conyza sumatrensis (Retz) Walk

PUBLICATION

J. Essent. Oil Res., Vol. 7, 83-84 (Jan/Feb 1995)

COMPOUNDS

43.70%	-	Lachnophyllum methyl ester
22.90%	-	Limonene
5.34%	-	Sabinene
5.25%	-	(E)-beta-Farnesene
4.98%	-	(E)-beta-Ocimene
4.81%	-	beta-Pinene
3.42%	-	isocaryophyllene
3.35%	-	aipha-Thujene
2.14%	-	Matricaria methyl ester
1.57%	-	gamma-Elemene
1.36%	-	Myrcene
1.13%	-	alpha-Muurolene
99.95	TOTAL %	12 COMPOUNDS

Coreopsis barteri leaf (Cameroon)

BC ΓANICAL SPECIES

Coreopsis barteri Oliv. & Hiern, fam. Asteraceae (Compositae)

AUTHOR

Menut,.C., et al.

TITLE

Aromatic Plants of Tropical Centra Africa. Part XXVl. Volatile Constituents of Leaves of Coreopsis barteri and C. grandiflora from Cameroon

PUBLICATION

Flavour Fragr. J., Vol. 11, 31-33 (1996)

COMPOUNDS

55.40%	-	Limonene
12.90%	-	alpna-Phellandrene
7.80%	-	Germacrene D
5.50%	-	Sabinene
2.50%	-	beta-Caryophyllene
2.30%	-	(E)-beta-Ocimene
2.10%	-	alpha-Pinene
1.80%	-	T-Muurolol
1.70%	-	alpha-Cadinol
1.60%	-	alpna-Humulene
1.30%	-	delta-Cadinene
1 00%	-	1, 8-Cineole
0.60%	-	alpha-Copaene
0.40%	-	Myrcene
0.40%	-	beta-Elemene
0.40%	-	beta-Cedrene

0.30%	-	alpha-Muurolene	
0.30%	-	gamma-Cadinene	
0.20%	-	Terpinen-4-ol	
0.05%	-	Camphene	
0.05%	-	beta-Pinene	
0.05%	-	gamma-Terpinene	
0.05%	-	Bicyclogermacrene	
98.70		TOTAL %	23 COMPOUNDS

Coreopsis grandiflora leaf (Cameroon)

BOTANICAL SPECIES

Coreopsis grandiflora Hogg ex Sweet, fam. Asteraceae (Compositae)

AUTHOR

Menut, C., et al.

TITLE

Aromatic Plants of Tropical Central Africa. Part XXVI. Volatile Constituents of Leaves of Coreopsis barteri and C. grandiflora from Cameroon

PUBLICATION

Flavour Fragr. J., Vol. 11, 31-33 (1996)

COMPOUNDS

42.10%	-	Germacrene D
11.70%	-	Myrcene
8.70%	-	alpha-Pinene
5.20%	-	1-Pnenylhepta-1, 3, 5-triyne
4.80%	-	beta-Farnesene
3.60%	-	T-Muurolol
3.10%	-	alpha-Cadinol
2.80%	-	Limonene
2.80%	-	delta-Cadinene
2.60%	-	Camphene
1.40%	-	beta-Caryophyllene
1.20%	-	beta-Pinene
1.20%	-	alpha-Cedrene
1.20%	-	Bicyclogermacrene
1.10%	-	beta-Copaene
1.00%	-	Bornyl acetate

1.00%	-	gamma-Cadinene	
0.90%	-	Precocene I	
0.80%	-	alpha-Humulene	
0.70%	-	beta-Elemene	
0.05%	-	Sabinene	
0.05%	-	alpha-Phellandrene	
0.05%	-	(E)-beta-Ocimene	
0.05%	-	gamma-Terpinene	
0.05%	-	Terpinen-4-ol	
0.05%	-	1, 8-Cineole	
0.05%	-	alpha-Copaene	
98.25		TOTAL %	27 COMPOUNDS

Dendranthema vestitum flower absolute (China)

BOTANICAL SPECIES

Dendranthema vestitum (Hemsl.) Ling ex Shih, fam, Asteraceae (Compositae)

AUTHOR

Liangfeng Zhu, Li Yonghua, Li Baoling, Lu Biyao & Xia Nianhe

TITLE

Aromatic Plants and Essential Constituents p. 95

PUBLICATION

South China Institute of Botany, Chinese Academy of Sciences, Hai Feng Publishing Co., Chinese National Node for APINMAP, distributed by Peace Book Co. Ltd., Hong Kong (1993)

COMPOUNDS

6.80%	-	1, 11-Dodecadiene
5.54%	-	Butyl tetradecanoate
4.50%	-	Oleic acid
4.39%	-	Camphor
3.64%	-	Longifolene
3.60%	-	beta-Caryophyllene
3.05%	-	Ethyl hexadecanoate
2.77%	-	Ethyldecanoate
2.66%	-	1, 8-Cineole
2.58%	-	Decanal
1.80%	-	Nerol
1.73%	-	Ethyl dodecanoate
1.61%	-	Chavicol
1.50%	-	Isoamyl undecanoate
1.43%	-	Ethyl tetradecanoate

1.39%	-	Terpinyl acetate (unknown isomer)
1.35%	-	Methyl palmitate
1.16%	-	Isobornyl acetate
1.07%	-	Linalool
0.82%	-	1-Octanol
0.81%	-	Octyl formate
0.75%	-	Methyl 2, 8-dimethylundecanoate
0.62%	-	Methyl decanoate
0.57%	-	alpha-Terpineol
0.53%	-	alpha-Copaene
0.49%	-	alpha-Hexylcinnamaldehyde (tent.)
0.46%	-	Trimethylpentadecane
0.46%	-	trans-Chrysanthenol
0.42%	-	Terpinen-4-ol
0.36%	-	Mayurone
0.32%	-	Isopropyl decanoate
0.30%	-	Isobomeol
0.26%	-	2, 3-Dicyclohexylbutae
0.26%	-	Heptadecanol-1
0.20%	-	Sabinene
0.16%	-	Tridecanal
0.15%	-	gamma-Patchoulene
0.14%	-	Borneol
0.06%	-	Camphene
0.05%	-	alpha-pinene
60.76		TOTAL % 40 COMPOUNDS

Egletes viscosa (flower heads)

BOTANICAL SPECIES

Egletes viscosa Less., fam. Asteraceae (Compositae)

AUTHOR

Craveiro, A.A., Alencar, J.W., Matos, F.J.A., and Machado, M.I.L.

TITLE

Essential Oil from Flower Heads of Egletes viscosa Less.

PUBLICATION

J. Essent. Oil Res., Vol. 4, 639-640 (Nov/Dec 1992)

COMPOUNDS

49.00%	-	trans-Pinocarvyl acetate
26.60%	-	beta-Pinene
6.50%	-	Myrtenyl acetate
2.70%	-	delta-3-Carene
2.00%	-	alpha-Pinene
1.10%	-	beta-Phellandrene
1.10%	-	Geranyl acetate
1.10%	-	trans-Pinocarveol
1.10%	-	Terpinen-4-yl acetate
0.70%	-	Myrcene
0.70%	-	alpha-Terpinyl acetate
0.50%	-	Pinocarvone
0.40%	-	alpha-Thujene
0.30%	-	Neryl acetate
0.30%	-	Myrtenol
0.30%	-	Neophytadiene
0.30%	-	cis-Carvyl acetate

0.20%	-	Terpinen-4-ol	
0.20%	-	Pinocamphone	
0.10%	-	alpha-Terpinene	
0.10%	-	Linalool	
0.10%	-	Borneol	
0.10%	-	alpha-Ylangene	
95.70		TOTAL %	23 COMPOUNDS

Erigeron Canadensis

BOTANICAL SPECIES

Erigeron canadensis L. [(Conyza canadensis (L.) Cronquist)], fam. Asteraceae

AUTHOR

Miyazawa, M., Yamamoto, K. and Kameoka, H.

TITLE

The Essential Oil of Erigeron canadensis L.

PUBLICATION

J. Essent. Oil Res., Vol. 4, 227-230 (May/Jun 1992)

COMPOUNDS

31.20%	-	Limonene
14.20%	-	Camphene
11.30%	-	Germacrene D
9.90%	-	cis-alpha-Bergamotene
7.60%	-	(E)-beta-Ocimene
7.20%	-	beta-Pinene
2.70%	-	Perillene
1.60%	-	(Z)-beta-Famesene
1.60%	-	(E)-beta-Farnesene
1.10%	-	alpha-Pinene
0.70%	-	ar-Curcumene
0.70%	-	(Z)-Nerolidol
0.60%	-	para-Cymene
0.40%	-	beta-Caryophyllene
0.30%	-	gamma-Terpinene
0.30%	-	Terpinolene
0.30%	-	alpha-Copaene

0.30%	-	alpha-Cedrerse
0.20%	-	(Z)-beta-Ocimene
0.20%	-	Nerol
0.20%	-	Geraniol
0.20%	-	delta-Cadinene
0.20%	-	beta-Cubebene
0.20%	-	beta-Sesquiphellandrene
0.10%	-	Spathulenol
0.10%	-	Cubenol
0.10%	-	delta-Cadinol
0.10%	-	alpha-Cadinol
0.10%	-	beta-Eudesmol
0.10%	-	beta-Ionone
0.01%	-	alpha-Terponeol
0.01%	-	alpha-Humulene
0.01%	-	Calamene
0.01%	-	alpha-Cubebene
0.01%	-	beta-Bourbonene
0.01%	-	beta-Curcumene
0.01%	-	alpha-Elemene
0.01%	-	Pentanal
0.01%	-	Ethyl formate
93.89		TOTAL % 39 COMPOUNDS

Eupatorium argentinum leaf

BOTANICAL SPECIES

Eupatorium argentinum Hook and Arn., fam Asteraceae (Compositae)

AUTHOR

Zygadio, J.A., Meastri, D.M., and Guzman, C.A.

TITLE

Comparative Study of the Essential Oils from Three Species of Eupatorium

PUBLICATION

Flavour Fragr. J., Vol. 11, 153-155 (1996)

COMPOUNDS

17.00%	-	alpha-Pinene
12.50%	-	para-Cymene
9.70%	-	Thymyl acetate
7.20%	-	beta-Caryophyllene
6.10%	-	beta-Pinene
4.10%	-	Carvacryl acetate
3.10%	-	alpha-Humulene
2.70%	-	alpha-Copaene
2.50%	-	delta-Cadinene
1.20%	-	Sabinene
1.20%	-	gamma-Muurolene
0.80%	-	Caryophyllene oxide
0.70%	-	Limonene
0.50%	-	Terpinen-4-ol
0.50%	-	alpha-Terpineol
0.50%	-	Carvacrol

0.40%	-	Neral	
0.30%	-	Geranial	
0.20%	-	Myrcene	
0.20%	-	Terpinolene	
0.10%	-	Thymol	
71.50		TOTAL %	21 COMPOUNDS

Eupatorium arnottianum leaf

BOTANICAL SPECIES

Eupatorium arnottianum Griseb., fam. Asteraceae (Compositae)

AUTHOR

Zydagio, J.A., et al.

TITLE

Analysis of the Essential Oil of the Leaves of Eupatorium arnottianum Griseb.

PUBLICATION

J. Essent. Oil Res., vol. 7, 677-678 (Nov/Dec 1995)

COMPOUNDS

30.00%	-	para-Cymene
13.70%	-	alpha-Pinene
12.32%	-	Thymyl acetate
11.70%	-	beta-Caryophyllene
5.26%	-	(Z)-beta-Ocimene
3.91%	-	beta-Pinene
2.11%	-	Carvacryl acetate
2.04%	-	gamma-Muurolene
1.84%	-	Cadinene (unknown isomer)
1.20%	-	alpha-Humulene
1.10%	-	alpha-Copaene
0.74%	-	Limonene
0.65%	-	Neral
0.61%	-	Sabinene
0.52%	-	Geranial
0.47%	-	Caryophyllene oxide

0.45%	-	Thymol	
0.27%	-	Terpinen-4-ol	
0.23%	-	Carvacrol	
0.21%	-	Myrcene	
0.16%	-	gamma-Terpinene	
0.14%	-	alpha-Terpineol	
0.12%	-	Terpinolene	
89.80		TOTAL %	23 COMPOUNDS

Eupatorium hecatanthum leaf

BOTANICAL SPECIES

Eupatorium hecatanthum (DC.) Baker, fam. Asteraceae (Compositae)

AUTHOR

Zygadio, J.A., Maestri, D.M., and Guzman, C.A.

TITLE

Comparative Study of the Essential Oils from Three Species of Eupatorium

PUBLICATION

Flavour Frag. J., Vol. 11, 153-155 (1996)

COMPOUNDS

13.40%	-	alpha-Pinene
10.60%	-	Thymyl acetate
8.10%	-	beta-Caryophyllene
7.80%	-	beta-Pinene
7.10%	-	Carvacrol
6.20%	-	beta-Ocimene
4,10%	-	Thymol
3.40%	-	Carvacryl acetate
3.30%	-	alpha-Copaene
3.10%	-	Limonene
3.00%	-	delta-Cadinene
2.30%	-	alpha-Humulene
1.80%	-	Myrcene
1.40%	-	gamma-Terpinene
1.20%	-	alpha-Muurolene
1.00%	-	Neral

1.00%	-	Geranial	
1.00%	-	Caryophyllene oxide	
0.50%	-	alpha-Terpineol	
0.40%	-	Terpinen-4-ol	
0.20%	-	Sabinene	
0.10%	-	Terpinolene	
81.00		TOTAL %	22 COMPOUNDS

Eupatorium maximilianii

BOTANICAL SPECIES

Eupatorium maximilianii (Erva de Sao Joao), fam. Asteraceae (Compositae)

AUTHOR

Maia, J.G.S., Ramos, L.S., Luz, A.I.R.,da Silva, M.L. and Zoghbi, M.d.G.B.

TITLE

Uncommon Brazilian Essential Oils of the Labiatae and Compositae

PUBLICATION

In: Flavors and Fragr.: a World Persp., Lawrence, B.M., Mookherjee, B.D., Willis,B.J. (Eds.),Proc. of the 10th Intern. Congress of Ess. Oils, Fragr. & Flavors, Washington, DC, USA,16-20 Nov.1986, Elsevier, Amsterdam (1988), 177-188

COMPOUNDS

13.24%	-	Germacrene B
10.45%	-	beta-Caryophyllene
6.24%	-	gamma-Elemene
6.03%	-	beta-Elemene
5.61%	-	alpha-Pinene
5.07%	-	Nerolidol (unknown isomer)
2.56%	-	Myrcene
2.66%	-	beta-Maaliene
2.40%	-	beta-Pinene
2.10%	-	delta-Cadinene
2.09%	-	alpha-Gurjunene
1.98%	-	(E)-beta-Ocimene
1.98%	-	alpha-Humulene

1.83%	-	Copaene (unknown isomer)
1.82%	-	Limonene
1.24%	-	Aromadendrene
1.19%	-	delta-Elemene
1.07%	-	beta-Bisabolene
1.00%	-	Sabinene
0.80%	-	gamma-Terpinene
0 63%	-	Terpinolene
0.52%	-	Germacrene A
0.37%	-	para-Cymene
0.34%	-	alpha-Phellandrene
0.30%	-	(Z)-beta-Ocimene
0.12%	-	delta-3-Carene
73.74		TOTAL % 26 COMPOUNDS

Eupatorium stoechadosmum

BOTANICAL SPECIES

Eupatorium stoechadosmum Hance, fam. Asteraceae (Compositae)

AUTHOR

Nguyen Xuan Dung et al.

TITLE

Composition of the Oil of Eupatorium stoechadosmum Hance from Vietnam

PUBLICATION

J. Essent. Oil Res., Vol. 3, 115-116 (Mar/Apr 1991)

COMPOUNDS

73.00%	-	Thymohydroquinone dimethylether
11.00%	-	Selina-3,7(11)-diene
8.90%	-	beta-Cafyophyllene
1.20%	-	beta-Elemene
0.50%	-	alpha-Selinene
0.40%	-	alpha-Humulene
0.40%	-	Caryophyllene oxide
0.30%	-	Methyl thymol
0.20%	-	beta-Pinene
0.20%	-	alpha-Terpinene
0.20%	-	Terpinen-4-ol
0.20%	-	1, 8-Cineole
0.20%	-	Methyl carvacrol
0.10%	-	alpha-Pinene
0.10%	-	Camphor
0.10%	-	beta-Selinene
0.01%	-	alpha-Phellandrene
97.01	TOTAL %	17 COMPOUNDS

Eupatorium subhastatum leaf

BOTANICAL SPECIES

Eupatorium subhastatum (DC.) Baker, fam. Asteraceae (Compositae)

AUTHOR

Zygadio, J.A., Maestri, D.M., and Guzman, C.A.

TITLE

Comparative Study of the Essential Oils from Three Species of Eupatorium

PUBLICATION

Flavour Fragr. J., Vol. 11, 153-155 (1996)

COMPOUNDS

24.80%	-	para-Cymene
11.00%	-	alpha-Pinene
5.90%	-	beta-Pinene
5.10%	-	alpha-Humulene
5.10%	-	alpha-Copaene
4.10%	-	delta-Cadinene
3.20%	-	Thymyl acetate
3.20%	-	Carvacryl acetate
1.60%	-	gamma-Muurolene
0.90%	-	Caryophyllene oxide
0.80%	-	Geranial
0.80%	-	Thymol
0.70%	-	Sabinene
0.70%	-	Limonene
0.70%	-	alpha-Terpineol
0.50%	-	beta-Caryophyllene

0.40%	-	Terpinen-4-ol	
0.30%	-	Carvacrol	
0.10%	-	Myrcene	
0.10%	-	Neral	
70.00		TOTAL %	20 COMPOUNDS

Grindela robusta

BOTANICAL SPECIES

Grindela robusta Nutt., fam. Asteraceae (Compositae)

AUTHOR

Kaitenbach, G., Schaefer, M. and Schimmer, O.

TITLE

Volatile Constituents of the Essential Oil of Grindela robusta Nutt. and Grindela squarrosa Dun.

PUBLICATION

J. Essent Oil Res., Vol. 5, 107-108 (Jan/Feb 1993)

COMPOUNDS

12.28%	-	Bornyl acetate
12.15%	-	alpha-Pinene
5.46%	-	Camphene
3.35%	-	Limonene
2.54%	-	beta-Pinene
2.27%	-	Borneol
0.88%	-	Myrcene
0.65%	-	Methyl eugenol
0.63%	-	beta-Caryophyllene
0.53%	-	para-Cymene
0.53%	-	Camphor
0.27%	-	Terpinolene
41.54	TOTAL %	12 COMPOUNDS

Grindela squarrosa

BOTANICAL SPECIES

Grindela squarrosa Dun., fam. Asteraceae (Compositae)

AUTHOR

Kaltenbach, G., Schaefer, M. and Schimmer, O.

TITLE

Volatile Constituents of the Essential Oil of Grindela robusta Nutt. and Grindela squarrosa Dun.

PUBLICATION

J. Essent. Oil Res., Vol. 5, 107-108 (Jan/Feb 1993)

COMPOUNDS

25.53%	-	alpha-Pinene
4.22%	-	Camphene
3.62%	-	Limonene
2.92%	-	beta-Caryophyllene
2.39%	-	beta-Pinene
1.53%	-	Borneol
1.35%	-	Bornyl acetate
1.24%	-	para-Cymene
0 78%	-	Terpinolene
0.59%	-	Camphor
0.36%	-	Myrcene
0.01%	-	Methyl eugenol
44.54	TOTAL %	12 COMPOUNDS

Helichrysum hypnoides (Madagascar)

BOTANICAL SPECIES

Helichrysum hypnoides, fam. Asteraceae (Compositae)

AUTHOR

Blanc, P.

TITLE

Composition of the oil of Helichrysum hynoides (3 samples)

PUBLICATION

Private communication Nov. 1993

COMPOUNDS

28.00%	-	beta-Caryophyllene
11.00%	-	Linalool
10.00%	-	1, 8-Cineole
5.00%	-	Limonene
4.00%	-	alpha-Humulene
2.20%	-	alpha-Pinene
2.00%	-	aipha-Terpineol
1.90%	-	Myrcene
1.50%	-	gamma-Terpinene
1.00%	-	alpha-Copaene
0.70%	-	beta-Pinene
0.50%	-	Camphene
0.50%	-	alpha-Terpinene
0.50%	-	Terpinolene
0.30%	-	para-Cymene
0.05%	-	Sabinene
69.15	TOTAL %	16 COMPOUNDS

Helichrysum odoratissimum

BOTANICAL SPECIES

Heiichrysum odoratissimum (L.) Less., fam. Asteraceae (Compositae)

AUTHOR

Lwande W., et al.

TITLE

Constituents of the Essential Oil of Helichrysum odoratissimum (L.) Less.

PUBLICATION

J. Essent. Oil Res., Vol. 5, 93-95 (1993)

COMPOUNDS

43.40%	-	alpha-Pinene
16.80%	-	(E, E)-Farnesol
14.60%	-	alpha-Humulene
8.20%	-	beta-Caryophyllene
4.90%.	-	Cedrol
3.40%	-	Citronellal
2.10%	-	Limonene
1.90%	-	Carvacrol
1.40%	-	1, 8-Cineole
0.60%	-	(E)-beta-Ocimene
0.60%	-	10-Nonadecanol
0.50%	-	para-Cymene
0.40%	-	Geraniol
0.30%	-	Myrcene
0.20%	-	Camphene
0.20%	-	Terpinolene
0.20%	-	Nonanal
0.20%	-	Nerol
0.20%	-	Linalyl acetate
100.10	TOTAL %	19 COMPOUNDS

Helichrysum bracteiferum (Madagascar)

BOTANICAL SPECIES

Helichrysym bracteiferum (Ramhiazina vavy), fam. Asteraceae (Compositae)

AUTHOR

Blanc, P.

TITLE

Composition of the oil of Helichrysum bracteuferum (2 samples)

PUBLICATION

Private communication Nov. 1993

COMPOUNDS

24.30%	-	1, 8-Cineole
11.20%	-	beta-Pinene
7.35%	-	alpha-Humulene
4.85%	-	beta-Caryophyllene
4.80%	-	alpha-Pinene
3.90%	-	Limonene
1.70%	-	Sabinene
1.40%	-	Linalool
1.30%	-	alpha-Terpineol
0.90%	-	Myrcene
0.80%	-	gamma-Terpinene
0.70%	-	alpha-Terpinene
0.70%	-	para-Cymene
0.45%	-	alpha-Copaene
0.35%	-	Terpinolene
0.10%	-	Camphene
64.80	TOTAL %	16 COMPOUNDS

Heterotheca inuloides leaf (Mexico)

BOTANICAL SPECIES

Heterotheca inuloides Cass., fam. Asteraceae (Compositae)

AUTHOR

Sagrero-Nieves, L, and Bartley, J.P.

TITLE

Volatile Components from the Leaves of Heterotheca inuloides Cass.

PUBLICATION

Flavour Fragr. J., Vol. 11, 49-51 (1996)

COMPOUNDS

22.50%	-	alpha-Cubebene
8.80%	-	Borneol
6.61%	-	Myrcene
6.58%	-	Caryophyllene oxide
6.10%	-	Bornyl acetate
5.58%	-	Camphor
5.00%	-	(E)-beta-Ocimene
4.57%	-	beta-Elemene
4.10%	-	Germacrene D
3.50%	-	beta-Bourbonene
3.13%	-	Limonene
3.10%	-	beta-Caryophyllene
3.02%	-	alpha-Cadinene
1.65%	-	beta-Pinene
1.60%	-	alpha-Terpineol
0.97%	-	Eugenol
0.58%	-	Benzaldehyde

0 52%	-	delta-Cadinene
0.47%	-	Menthone
0.40%	-	alpha-Curcumene
0.34%	-	Sabinene
0.32%	-	gamma-Terpinene
0.27%	-	alpha-Pinene
0.26%	-	alpha-Bergamotene
0.23%	-	1, 4-Cineole
0.22%	-	cis-Sabinene hydrate
0.21%	-	beta-Phellandrene
0.17%	-	Terpinolene
0.16%	-	alpha-Terpinene
0.15%	-	alpha-Humulene
0.12%	-	Anethole
0.11%	-	(E)-Nerolidol
0.11%	-	Benzyl alcohol
0.10%	-	(Z)-beta-Ocimene
0.08%	-	Linalool
0.05%	-	Geranyl acetate
0.04%	-	gamma-Muurolene
0.03%	-	para-Cymene
0.03%	-	Carvone
0.02%	-	Geraniol
0.02%	-	Cadalene
0.02%	-	(E)-2-Hexenol
91.84	TOTAL %	42 COMPOUNDS

Ichtyothere terminalis (Brazil)

BOTANICAL SPECIES

Ichtyothere terminalis (common name: Mata-peixe or cunabi), fam. Asteraceae

AUTHOR

Maia, J.G.S., Ramos, L.S., Luz, A.I.R., da Silva, M.L., and Zoghbi, M.d.G.B.

TITLE

Uncommon Brazilian Essential Oils of the Labiatae and Compositae

PUBLICATION

in: Flavors and Fragr.: a World Persp., Lawrence, B.M., Mookherjee, B.D., Willis, B.J. (Eds.), Proc. of the 10th Intern. Congress of Ess. Oils, Fragr. & Flavors, Washington, DC, USA.16-20 Nov.1986, Elsevier, Amsterdam (1988), 177-188

COMPOUNDS

35.83%	-	Limonene
19.84%	-	alpha-Pinene
14.83%	-	Sabinene
5 30%	-	delta-3-Carene
1.90%	-	trans-Pinocarveol
1.77%	-	Carvone
1.72%	-	Camphene
1.02%	-	Copaene (unknown isomer)
0.99%	-	Myrcene
0.84%	-	Verbenone
0.83%	-	Methyl chavicol
0.73%	-	delta-Cadinene
0.71%	-	garnma-Terpinene

0.71%	-	Terpinen-4-ol	
0.68%	-	para-Cymene	
0.46%	-	gamma-Muurolene	
0.40%	-	beta-Caryophyllene	
0.39%	-	Terpinolene	
0.38%	-	trans-Carveol	
0.27%	-	Linalool	
0.24%	-	alpha-Terpinene	
89.84		TOTAL %	21 COMPOUNDS

Inula viscosa (Turkey)

BOTANICAL SPECIES

Inula viscosa (L) Aiton (Dittrichia viscosa (L.) Greuter), fam.Asteraceae

AUTHOR

Perez-Alonso, M.-J., et al.

TITLE

Composition of the Volatile Oil from the Aerial Parts of Inula Viscosa (L.) Aiton

PUBLICATION

Flavour Fragr. J, Vol. 11, 349-351 (1996)

COMPOUNDS

34.00%	-	Bornyl acetate
23.00%	-	Borneol
11.40%	-	Isobornyl acetate
2.80%	-	Caryophylladienols
2.30%	-	beta-Pinene
1.10%	-	Caryophyllene oxide
1.10%	-	(E)-Nerolidol
1.00%	-	beta-Caryophyllene
1.00%	-	Eudesmols (unknown isomer)
0.70%	-	Artemisia ketone
0.60%	-	alpha-Pinene
0.60%	-	p-Cymen-8-ol
0.60%	-	beta-Eudesmol
0.50%	-	Myrcene
0.50%	-	Nerolidyl acetate
0.45%	-	Camphene hydrate

0.40%	-	T-Cadinol
0.35%	-	Camphor
0.35%	-	Germacrene D
0.30%	-	Terpinen-4-ol
0.30%	-	dehydro-1, 8-Cineole
0.25%	-	Camphene
0.25%	-	Linalool
0.20%	-	alpha-Humulene
0.20%	-	trans-Verbenol
0.20%	-	Isobomeol
0.15%	-	Limonene
0.15%	-	1, 8-Cineole
0.15%	-	beta-Sellnene
0.15%	-	Yomogi alcohol
0.15%	-	beta-Damascenone
0.10%	-	delta-3-Carene
0.10%	-	para-Cymene
0.10%	-	alpha-Muurolene
0.10%	-	gamma-Cadinene
0.10%	-	alpha-Fenchol
0.10%	-	Artemisia alcohol
0.10%	-	Bornyl formate
0.05%	-	(E)-beta-Ocimene
0.05%	-	Terpinolene
0.05%	-	alpha-Terpineol
0.05%	-	alpha-Copaene
0.05%	-	beta-Bourbonene
0.05%	-	beta-Fenchol
0.05%	-	beta-Calacorene
0.01%	-	alpha-Thujene
0.01%	-	Sabinene
0.01%	-	alpha-Phellandrene

0.01%	-	alpha-Terpinene	
0.01%	-	(Z)-beta-Ocimene	
0.01%	-	Carvacrol	
0.01%	-	cis-Calamenene	
86.32		TOTAL %	52 COMPOUNDS

Pectis prostrata leaf

BOTANICAL SPECIES

Pectis prostrata Cav., fam. Asteraceae (Compositae)

AUTHOR

Pino, J.A., Rosado, A., and Fuentes, V.

TITLE

Chemical Composition of the Leaf Oil of Pectis prostrata Cav. from Cuba

PUBLICATION

J. Essent. Oil Res., Vol. 8, 579-580 (Sep/Oct 1996)

COMPOUNDS

70.74%	-	Perillaldehyde
16.20%	-	Limonene
3.63%	-	Perillyl alcohol
1.73%	-	Sabinene
0.91%	-	1-Octanol
0.65%	-	1-Decanol
0.60%	-	alpha-Pinene
0.48%	-	Thymol
0.39%	-	alpha-Humulene
0.37%	-	Terpinen-4-ol
0.31%	-	Myrcene
0.24%	-	gamma-Terpinene
0.18%	-	(E)-beta-Ocimene
0.16%	-	para-Cymene
0.12%	-	alpha-Thujene
0.09%	-	Linalool
0.09%	-	Humulene oxide

0.07%	-	Camphene
0.07%	-	Carvone
0.06%	-	Terpinolene
0.05%	-	Caryophyila-3,8(13)-dien-5,alpha-ol
0.04%	-	beta-Elemene
0.02%	-	beta-Caryophyllene
0.02%	-	trans-Linalool oxide (5) (furanoid)
97.22	TOTAL %	24 COMPOUNDS

Psiadia lithospermifolia

BOTANICAL SPECIES

Psiadia Iithospermifolia (Lam.) Cordem., fam. Asteraceae (Compositae)

AUTHOR

Gurib-Fakim, A., Bourrel, C., Kodja, H., and Govinden, J.

TITLE

Chemical Composition of the Essential Oils of Psidia lithospermifolia (Lam.) Cordem. and P. viscosa (Lam.) A.J. Scott of the Asteraceae Family

PUBLICATION

J. Essent. Oil Res., Vol. 7, 535-535 (Sep/Oct 1995)

COMPOUNDS

51.55%	-	alpha-Asarone
8.12%	-	(E)-beta-Farnesene
5.15%	-	delta-Elemene
4.80%	-	4(l4), 7(11)-Selinadiene
3.69%	-	delta-Selinene
2.20%	-	(E, Z)-alpha-Famesene
1.85%	-	gamma-Cadinene
1.84%	-	alpha-Cedrene
1.71%	-	ar-Curcumene
1.59%	-	beta-Bisabolene
0.94%	-	gamma-Elemene
0.87%	-	alpha-Humulene
84.32	TOTAL %	12 COMPOUNDS

Psiadia viscosa

BOTANICAL SPECIES

Psiadia viscosa (Lam.) A.J. Scott, fam. Asteraceae (Compositae)

AUTHOR

Gurib-Fakim, A., Bourrel, C., Kodia, H., and Govinden, J.

TITLE

Chemical Composition of the Essential Oils of Psiadia lithospermifolia (Lam.) Cordem. and P. viscosa (Lam.) A.J. Scott of the Asteraceae Family

PUBLICATION

J. Essent. Oil Res., Vol. 7, 533-535 (Sep/Oct 1995)

COMPOUNDS

25.86%	-	Pentyl 4-isopropylbenzoate
13.35%	-	alpha-Asarone
7.50%	-	Guaiol
7.50%	-	alpha-Patchoulene
7.45%	-	Calarene
5.30%	-	gamma-Cadinene
4.20%	-	beta-Patohoulene
3.00%	-	beta-Cedrene
2.50%	-	Cadina-1, 4-diene
2.40%	-	Methyl eugenol
1.94%	-	Agarospirol
1.68%	-	4(14), 7(11)-Selinadiene
1.15%	-	beta-Himachalene
1.10%	-	Terpinen-4-ol
1.05%	-	Aristolone
0.30%	-	alpha-Terpineol

0.17%	-	alpha-Terpinene	
0.14%	-	Linalool	
0.12%	-	alpha-Phellandrene	
0.10%	-	alpha-Thujene	
86.81		TOTAL %	20 COMPOUNDS

Pteronia incana 1

BOTANICAL SPECIES

Pteronia incana, fam. Asteraceae (Compositae)

AUTHOR

Bruns, K., and Meiertoberens, M.

TITLE

Volatile Constituents of Pteronia incana (Compositae) (monoterpene fraction)

PUBLICATION

Flavour Fragr. J., Vol. 2, (4), 157-162 (1987)

COMPOUNDS

32.50%	-	beta-Pinene	
18.60%	-	alpha-Pinene	
11.30%	-	para-Cymene	
10.30%	-	Myrcene	
9.00%	-	1, 8-Cineole	
7.40%	-	Sabinene	
7.00%	-	Limonene	
0.90%	-	(E)-beta-Ocimene	
0.40%	-	alpha-Phellandrene	
0.20%	-	alpha-Terpinene	
0.10%	-	Terpinolene	
97.70		TOTAL %	11 COMPOUNDS

Pteronia incana 2

BOTANICAL SPECIES

Pteronia incana, fam. Asteraceae (Compositae)

AUTHOR

Bruns, K., and Meiertoberens, M.

TITLE

Volatile Constituents of Pteronia incana (Compositae) (sesquiterpene fraction)

PUBLICATION

Flavour Fragr. J., Vol. 2, (4), 157-162 (1987)

COMPOUNDS

7.20%	-	Methyl eugenol
5.30%	-	Terpinen-4-ol
3.20%	-	beta-Caryophyllene
2.30%	-	delta-Cadinene
2.10%	-	ar-Curcumene
1.95%	-	1, 8-Cineole
1.30%	-	alpha-Terpineol
1.30%	-	trans-Pinocarveol
1.20%	-	alpha-Humulene
1.20%	-	Bicyclogermacrene
1.10%	-	Muurolene(s) (unknown structure)
0.90%	-	Linalool
0.80%	-	alpha-Terpinyl acetate
0.80%	-	p-Cymen-8-ol
0.70%	-	Myrtenol
0.70%	-	alpha-Calacorene
0.50%	-	Myrtenal

0.50%	-	Cuminaldehyde
0.40%	-	delta-Terpineol
0.30%	-	Geranylacetone
0.30%	-	trans-Carveol
0.30%	-	alpha-Cadinene
0.30%	-	Methyl hexanoate
0.30%	-	cis-Sabinol
0.20%	-	cis-Carveol
0.20%	-	Ethyl hexanoate
0.20%	-	trans-Myrtanol
0.10%	-	alpha-Fenchol
0.10%	-	(-)-Isopulegol
0.10%	-	Isoamyl isobutyrate
0.10%	-	trans-Sabinol
0.10%	-	Myrtenyl acetate
36.05	TOTAL %	32 COMPOUNDS

Santolina chamaecyparissus (France) 1

BOTANICAL SPECIES

Santolina chamaecyparissus L, fam. Asteraceae (Compositae)

AUTHOR

Derbesy, M., Touche, J., and Zola, A.

TITLE

The Essential Oil of Santolina chamaecyparissus L. (average of three analyses; trace = 0.5%)

PUBLICATION

J. Ess. Oil Res., Vol. 1, 269-275, (Nov./Dec. 1989)

COMPOUNDS

32.50%	-	Artemisia ketone
12.50%	-	beta-Phellandrene
11.50%	-	Myrcene
4.00%	-	Sabinene
4.00%	-	beta-Pinene
1.05%	-	Terpinolene
1.00%	-	Limonene
1.00%	-	1, 8-Cineole
1.00%	-	Yomogi alcohol
0.95%	-	Camphor
0.75%	-	Camphene
0.75%	-	Artemisia alcohol
0.40%	-	alpha-Pinene
0.05%	-	alpha-Phellandrene
0.05%	-	alpha-Terpinene
0.05%	-	para-Cymene
0.05%	-	gamma-Terpinene

0.05%	-	Borneol	
0.05%	-	Terpinen-4-ol	
0.05%	-	Sabinene hydrate	
0.05%	-	Artemisiatriene	
71.80		TOTAL%	21 COMPOUNDS

Santolina chamaecyparissus (France) 2

BOTANICAL SPECIES

Santolina chamaecyparissus L, fam. Asteraceae (Compositae)

AUTHOR

Vernin, G.

TITLE

Volatile Constituents of the Essential Oil of Santolina chamaecyparissus L.

PUBLICATION

J. Ess. Oil Res., Vol. 3, 49-53 (Jan/Feb. 1991)

COMPOUNDS

45.00%	-	Artemisia ketone
15.00%	-	Myrcene
5.50%	-	Sabinene
5.00%	-	beta-Phellandrene
4.70%	-	beta-Pinene
3.00%	-	Camphene
2.00%	-	1, 8-Cineole
1.50%	-	Limonene
1.50%	-	Borneol
1.50%	-	Camphor
1.50%	-	Artemisia alcohol
1.30%	-	Yomogi alcohol
1.00%	-	alpha-Thujene
0.60%	-	Linalyl acetate
0.50%	-	para-Cymene
0.50%	-	2-Propylfuran
0.50%	-	3, 3, 5-Trimethylcyclohexanone

0.40% - Terpinen-4-ol
0.25% - Perillene
0.20% - Linalool
0.20% - Camphene hydrate
0.15% - Aromadendrene
0.10% - gamma-Terpinene
0.10% - Neral
0.10% - m-Methylethylbenzene
0.10% - Trimethylbenzene (unknown structure)
0.08% - Cuminaldehyde
0.06% - Azulene
0.05% - alpha-Terpineol
0.05% - 1, 5-Menthadienol-7
0.05% - l-Ethyl-2-methylbenzene
0.05% - p-Methylethylbenzene
0.05% - 1, 2-Dimethyl-3-(1 methylethenyl)cyclopentanol
0.04% - p-Cymen-8-ol
0.04% - beta-Bourbonene
0.04% - Methyl carvacrol
0.04% - p-Menthatriene (isomer)
0.04% - 1-Methylnaphthalene
0.03% - Carvone
0.03% - Myrtenal
0.03% - 2-Pentylfuran
0.03% - Germacrene D
0.03% - Campholene aldehyde
0.03% - Dihydrocarvone
0.03% - Nopinone
0.03% - 1, 3, 5-Trimethylbenzene
0.03% - Tetramethylbenzene (unknown structure)

0.03%	-	Caranol
0.02%	-	(Z)-beta-Ocimene
0.02%	-	Bornyl acetate
0.02%	-	Geranyl acetate
0.02%	-	Germacrene B
0.02%	-	Isopinocamphone
0.02%	-	4-Methylacetophenone
0.01%	-	alpha-Pinene
0.01%	-	alpha-Terpinene
0.01%	-	(E)-beta-Ocimene
0.01%	-	Terpinolene
0.01%	-	beta-Selinene
0.01%	-	beta-Farnesene
0.01%	-	2-Decenal
0.01%	-	alpha-Farnesene
0.01%	-	(Z)-3-Hexenol
0.01%	-	(Z)-3-Hexenal
0.01%	-	(E)-2-Hexenyl acetate
0.01%	-	Isoamyl 2-methylbutyrate
0.01%	-	p-Xylene
0.01%	-	N.N-Dimethylformamide
0.01%	-	(Z)-2-Hexenyl acetate
0.01%	-	2-Methylnaphthalene
0.01%	-	5-Methylhexanal
0.01%	-	1, 3-Dimethyl-2-ethylbenzene
0.01%	-	2-Butylcyclopent-2-en-1-one
93.40	TOTAL %	73 COMPOUNDS

Pectis elongata

BOTANICAL SPECIES

Pectis elongata Kunth, fam. Asteraceae (Compositae)

AUTHOR

Prudent, D., Perineau, F., Bessiere, J.M., and Michel, G.

TITLE

Analysis of the Essential Oil of Pectis elongata Kunth from Martinique. Evaluation of Its Bacteriostatic and Fungistatic Properties (3 sitesampl.)

PUBLICATION

J. Essent. Oil Res., Vol. 7, 63-68 (Jan/Feb 1995)

COMPOUNDS

30.00%	-	Geranial
20.00%	-	Neral
10.00%	-	Geranic acid
4.00%	-	Neryl acid
2.00%	-	Geraniol
2.00%	-	1-Tridecene
1.30%	-	Linalool
1.00%	-	Nerol
1.00%	-	cis-Linalool oxide (unknown isomer)
1.00%	-	Humulene oxide II
0.75%	-	1-Undecene
0.50%	-	Limonene
0.50%	-	Neryl acetate
0.50%	-	Geranyl acetate
0.50%	-	6-Methyl-5-hepten-2-one
0.30%	-	Piperitone

0.30%	-	cis-Linalool oxide (5) (furanoid)	
0.20%	-	trans-Linalool oxide (5) (furanoid)	
0.10%	-	delta-Cadinene	
0.01%	-	beta-Patchoulene	
75.96		TOTAL %	20 COMPOUNDS

Santolina chamaecyparissus (France) 3

BOTANICAL SPECIES

Santolina chamaecyparissus L, fam. Asteraceae (Compositae)

AUTHOR

Brunke, E.J., Hammerschmidt, F.-J., and G. Schmaus

TITLE

The Essential Oil of Santolina Chamaecyparissus L. (average of 2 samples from Fa. Adrian, Marseille, France)

PUBLICATION

Dragoco Report, Vol. 39 (4), 151-167 (1992)

COMPOUNDS

32.11%	-	Artemisia ketone
16.62%	-	beta-Phellandrene
9.25%	-	Longiverbenone
7.93%	-	Myrcene
4.63%	-	Sabinene
4.40%	-	beta-Pinene
1.90%	-	Terpinolene
1.81%	-	gamma-Curcumene
1.75%	-	Camphor
1.50%	-	Limonene
1.50%	-	ar-Curcumene
1.34%	-	alpha-Longipinene
1.21%	-	Artemisia alcohol
1 14%	-	Germacrene D
0.90%	-	Borneol
0.82%	-	(E)-Anethole
0.75%	-	Bicyclogermacrene
0.71%	-	Spathulenol
0.65%	-	alpha-Pinene

0.63%	-	Yomogi alcohol
0.62%	-	Camphene
0.54%	-	Cryptone
0.46%	-	Caryophyllene oxide
0.43%	-	Ipsenone
0.37%	-	para-Cymene
0.34%	-	tras-Chrysanthenol
0.30%	-	Terpien-4-ol
0.28%	-	gamma-Terpinene
0.28%	-	Aromadendrene
0.22%	-	alpha-Phellandrene
0.17%	-	alpha-Terpinene
0.16%	-	Linalool
0.15%	-	p-Cymen-8-ol
0.15%	-	Cuminaldehyde
0.14%	-	Myrtenal
0.13%	-	Longiverbenol
0.12%	-	delta-Cadinene
0.11%	-	trans-Sabinene hydrate
0.11%	-	Myrtenol
0.09%	-	alpha-Ylangene
0.08%	-	Methyl thymol
0.07%	-	Cumin alcohol
0.06%	-	cis-Sabinene hydrate
0.05%	-	Bornyl acetate
0.05%	-	beta-Elemene
0.05%	-	T-Cadinol
0.04%	-	trans-p-Mentri-2-en-1-ol
0.02%	-	Piperitone
0.01%	-	1, 8-Cineole
0.01%	-	gamma-Cadinene
97.16		TOTAL % 50 COMPOUNDS

Santolina chamaecyparissus (Egypt)

BOTANICAL SPECIES

Santolina chamaecyparissus L, fam. Asteraceae (Compositae)

AUTHOR

Aboutabl, E.A., Hammerschmidt, F.J., and Elazzouny, A.A.

TITLE

The essential oil of Santolina chamaecyparissus L.

PUBLICATION

Sci. Pharm., Vol. 55, 267-271 (1987)

COMPOUNDS

44.50%	-	Artemisia ketone
15.10%	-	Camphor
2.90%	-	Camphene
2.80%	-	beta-Pinene
2.80%	-	beta-Phellandrene
2.10%	-	alpha-Bisabolol
1.80%	-	Myrcene
1.60%	-	Sabinene
1.50%	-	Yomogi alcohol
1.50%	-	ar-Curcumene
1.40%	-	Santolinatriene
0.83%	-	Cryptone
0.79%	-	Borneol
0.66%	-	Limonene
0.59%	-	2, 6-Dimethyl-2, 7-octadien-4-ol
0.54%	-	Terpinen-4-ol
0.47%	-	4-Methylacetophenone
0.43%	-	para-Cymene

0.42% - p-Cymen-8-ol

0.41% - Irans-Pinocarveol

0.37% - (E)-Nerolidol

0.34% - beta-Elemene

0.33% - Caryophyllene oxide

0.32% - Spathulenol

0.32% - Germacrene D

0.30% - 2-Methyl-2-propenal

0.27% - gamma-Terpinene

0.26% - Terpinolene

0.26% - Myrtenol

0.26% - Cuminaldehyde

0.26% - alpha-Bisabolol oxide B

0.19% - Pinocarvone

0.18% - alpha-Terpineol

0.14% - Cumin alcohol

0.13% - alpha-Pinene

0.11% - alpha-Terpinene

0.11% - Myrtenal

0.10% - 2-Methylbenzyl butyrate

0.08% - alpha, p-Dimethylstyrene

0.07% - alpha-Cadinol

0.07% - Perillyl alcohol

0.06% - Perillene

0.06% - Santolina alcohol

0.06% - Methylnaphthalene (unknown structure)

0.05% - Hexanal

0.04% - beta-Farnesene

0.04% - 6-Methyl-5-hepten-2-one

0.04% - Benzyl pentanoate

0.03% - Isoamyl isovalerate

0.01%	-	alpha-Phellandrene	
0.01%	-	Bornyl acetate	
0.01%	-	trans-Sabinene hydrate	
0.01%	-	2-Pentylfuran	
0.01%	-	2-Methylbutanol	
0.01%	-	1-Pentanol	
0.01%	-	2-Methylfuran	
0.01%	-	2-Butanone	
88.07		TOTAL %	57 COMPOUNDS

Santolina neapolitana (Italy)

BOTANICAL SPECIES

Santolina neapolitana Jordan et Fourr., fam. Asteraceae (Compositae)

AUTHOR

Senatore, F. & V. De Feo

TITLE

Composition of the Essential Oils of Santolina neapolitana Jordan et Fourr.

PUBLICATION

Flavour Fragr. J., Vol. 9, 77-79 (1994)

COMPOUNDS

31.90%	-	gamma-Muurolene
15.50%	-	alpha-Pinene
9.40%	-	Borneol
4.70%	-	Bornyl acetate
3.40%	-	Germacrene B
2.80%	-	delta-Cadinol
2.70%	-	beta-Pinene
2.70%	-	T-Muurolol
2.60%	-	Pinocarvone
2.00%	-	Camphene
1.90%	-	Nerolidol (unknown isomer)
1.80%	-	Bisabolol (unknown isomer)
1.70%	-	Terpinen-4-ol
1.70%	-	Camphor
1.70%	-	Opiopenone (unknown isomer)
1.40%	-	trans-Sabinene hydrate

1.40%	-	(Z)-beta-Farnesene
1.20%	-	beta-Caryophyllene
1.20%	-	beta-Farnesene
1.10%	-	Sesquiterpene alcohols (unknown)
1.00%	-	delta-Cadinene
0.80%	-	Myrcene
0.70%	-	1, 8-Cineole
0.60%	-	alpha-Muurolene
0.50%	-	Sesquiterpene hydrocarbons (unknown)
0.50%	-	trans-Calamenene
0.40%	-	gamma-Terpinene
0.40%	-	alpha-Copaene
0.40%	-	beta-Gurjunene
0.20%	-	Sabinene
0.20%	-	Verbenone
0.20%	-	Isoborneol
0.10%	-	alpha-Phellandrene
0.10%	-	alpha-Terpinene
0.10%	-	para-Cymene
0.10%	-	Limonene
0.10%	-	Ylangene
0.10%	-	Dihydrocarveol
0.10%	-	iso-Dihydrocarveol
0.05%	-	delta-3-Carene
0.05%	-	Artemisia alcohol
0.05%	-	Verbenol
0.05%	-	cis-Calamenene
99.60		TOTAL % 43 COMPOUNDS

Santolina pectina

BOTANICAL SPECIES

Santolina pectina Lag., fam. Asteraceae (Compositae)

AUTHOR

Perez Alonso, M.J., and Velasco Nequeruela, A.

TITLE

The Essential Oils of Four Santolina Species

PUBLICATION

Flavour Fragr. J., Vol. 3, (1), 37-42 (1988)

COMPOUNDS

12.40%	-	beta-Eudesmol
9.30%	-	alpha-Cadinol
6.90%	-	delta-Cadinol
4.60%	-	gamma-Eudesmol
4.30%	-	beta-Elemol
3.90%	-	Ledol
2.60%	-	Spathulenol
2.60%	-	ar-Curcumene
2.60%	-	(Z)-Nerolidol
2.40%	-	delta-Cadinene
2.40%	-	Farnesol (unknown isomer)
2.30%	-	Oplopenone (unknown isomer)
2.00%	-	(1R,5R,9S)-Caryophylla-4(12),8(13)-dien-5, alpha-ol
2.00%	-	Campherenone
1.80%	-	1, 8-Cineole
1.60%	-	Copaenol
1.40%	-	alpha-Pinene

1.40%	-	alpha-Bisabolene
1.40%	-	Caryophyllene oxide
1.30%	-	Eugenyl acetate
1.20%	-	Terpinolene
1.20%	-	Terpinen-4-ol
1.20%	-	beta-Caryophyllene
1.10%	-	beta-Pinene
0.80%	-	Borneol
0.80%	-	Elemene (unknown isomer)
0.80%	-	gamma-Terpineol
0.50%	-	Sabinene
0.50%	-	Myrcene
0.50%	-	Isolongifolene oxide
0.40%	-	Limonene
0.40%	-	beta-Terpineol
0.30%	-	gamma-Terpinene
0.20%	-	alpha-Terpinene
0.10%	-	alpha-Terpineol
0.10%	-	Artemisia ketone
0.07%	-	3, 3, 6-Trimethyl-1,4-heptadien-6-ol
0.04%	-	Camphor
0.04%	-	trans-Verbenol
0.03%	-	Citronellal
0.03%	-	trans-Pinocarveol
79.51	TOTAL %	41 COMPOUNDS

Santolina canescens

BOTANICAL SPECIES

Santolina rosmarinifolia (L.) ssp. canescens (Lag.) Nyman, fam. Asteraceae

AUTHOR

Perez-Alonso, M.J., and velasco Negueruela, A.

TITLE

The Essential Oils of Four Santolina Species.

PUBLICATION

Flavour Fragr. J., vol. 3, (1), 37-42 (1988)

COMPOUNDS

15.00%	-	Camphor
11.60%	-	1, 8-Cineole
9.90%	-	beta-Pinene
8.60%	-	beta-Eudesmol
7.40%	-	ar-Curcumene
6.50%	-	Myrcene
5.50%	-	Sabinene
3.50%	-	Terpinen-4-ol
3.20%	-	Farnesol (unknown isomer)
2.10%	-	gamma-Terpinene
1.80%	-	Spathulenol
1.80%	-	(Z)-Nerolidol
1.70%	-	Borneol
1.60%	-	Oplopenone (unknown isomer)
1.20%	-	alpha-Pinene
1.20%	-	alpha-Terpinene
1.10%	-	delta-Cadinol

0.80%	-	Terpinolene
0.80%	-	delta-Cadinene
0.80%	-	Elemene (unknown isomer)
0.70%	-	Limonene
0.70%	-	cis-Sabinene hydrate
0.70%	-	Ledol
0.70%	-	gamma-Terpineol
0.70%	-	Copaenol
0.70%	-	(1R, 5R, 9S)-Caryophylla-4(12), 8(13)-dien-5, alpha-ol
0.50%	-	alpha-Terpineol
0.50%	-	beta-Elemol
0.40%	-	Eugenyl acetate
0.20%	-	beta-Caryophyllene
0.20%	-	alpha-Bisabolene
0.20%	-	beta-Terpineol
0.10%	-	Safrole
0.10%	-	3, 6, 6-Trimethylbicyclo [3.1.0] hexane-3 carboxaldehyde
0.04%	-	trans-verbenol
0.03%	-	Citronellal
0.03%	-	trans-Piocarveol
92.60	TOTAL %	37 COMPOUNDS

Santolina rosmarinifolia

BOTANICAL SPECIES

Santolina rosmarinifolia L.ssp.rosmarinifolia, fam.Asteraceae (Compositae)

AUTHOR

Perez Alonso, M.J., and Velasco Negueruela A.

TITLE

The Essential Oils of Four Santolina Species

PUBLICATION

Flavour Fragr. J., Vol. 3, (1), 37-42 (1988)

COMPOUNDS

13.40%	-	beta-Eudesmol
8.90%	-	beta-Pinene
8.90%	-	1, 8-Cineole
7.80%	-	Myrcene
6.60%	-	Sabinene
5.80%	-	ar-Curcumene
2.40%	-	delta-Cadinol
2.00%	-	Terpinen-4-ol
1.90%	-	alpha-Terpineol
1.80%	-	Copaenol
1.60%	-	Ledol
1.50%	-	delta-Cadinene
1.50%	-	gamma-Eudesmol
1.40%	-	Spathulenol
1.40%	-	(Z)-Nerolidol
1.40%	-	Oplopenone (unknown isomer)
1.30%	-	Eugenyl acetate

1.20%	-	Borneol
1.10%	-	Camphor
1.10%	-	Elemene (unknown isomer)
1.00%	-	alpha-Pinene
0.90%	-	Limonene
0.80%	-	alpha-Terpinene
0.80%	-	beta-Elemol
0.70%	-	cis-Sabinene hydrate
0.60%	-	Campherenone
0.55%	-	Safrote
0.55%	-	3, 6, 6-Trimethylbicyclo [3.1.0] hexane-3 carboxaldehyde
0.50%	-	beta-Caryophyllene
0.50%	-	Guaiacol
0.30%	-	gamma-Terpinene
0.30%	-	Terpinolene
0.30%	-	Caryophyllene oxide
0.20%	-	beta-Terpineol
81.00		TOTAL % . 34 COMPOUNDS

Santolina semidentata

BOTANICAL SPECIES

Santolina semidentata Hoffmanns. & Link, fam. Asteraceae (Compositae)

AUTHOR

Perez Alonso, MJ., and Velasco Negueruela, A.

TITLE

The Essential Oils of Four Santolina Species

PUBLICATION

Flavour, Fragr. J, Vol. 3, (1), 37-42 (1988)

COMPOUNDS

6.40%	-	beta-Eudesmol
4.90%	-	alpha-Cadinol
3.00%	-	alpha-Pinene
2.70%	-	Isolongifolene oxide
2.50%	-	(Z)-Nerolidol
2.40%	-	Spathulenol
2.40%	-	beta-Terpineol
2.20%	-	ar-Curcumene
2.10%	-	delta-Cadinene
1.90%	-	Borneol
1.80%	-	beta-Pinene
1.80%	-	Limonene
1.80%	-	1, 8-Cineole
1.80%	-	gamma-Terpineol
1.80%	-	Copaenol
1.70%	-	Campherenone
1.50%	-	Myrcene

1.50%	-	gamma-Eudesmol
1.50%	-	(1R, 5R, 9S) -Caryophylla-4(12), 8(13)-dien 5, alpha-ol
1.40%	-	Elemene (unknown isomer)
1.30%	-	Sabinene
1.30%	-	Terpinen-4-ol
1.30%	-	beta-Caryophyllene
1.30%	-	Caryophyllene oxide
1.20%	-	Eugenyl acetate
1.20%	-	Oplopenone (unknown isorner)
1.10%	-	alpha-Bisabolene
1.10%	-	cis-Sabinene hydrate
1.00%	-	Guaiacol
0.90%	-	beta-Elemol
0.80%	-	alpha-Terpineol
0.70%	-	alpha-Terpinene
0.70%	-	Citroellal
0.50%	-	trans-Pinocarveol
0.50%	-	trans-Verbenol
0.40%	-	Terpinolene
0.40%	-	Camphor
0.40%	-	3, 3, 6-Trimethyl-1, -heptadien-6-ol
0.30%	-	gamma-Terpinene
0.20%	-	Artemisia ketone
63.70		TOTAL % 40 COMPOUNDS

Senecio

BOTANICAL SPECIES

Senecio glaucus ssp. coronopifolius (Maire Alexander), fam. Asteraceae

AUTHOR

Pooter de, H.L. et al.

TITLE

The volatile Fraction of Senecio giaucus subsp. Coronopifolius

PUBLICATION

Flavour, Fragr. J., Voi. 1, (4&5), 159-163 (1986)

COMPOUNDS

23.70%	-	Myrcene
21.30%	-	dehydro-Fukinone
9.90%	-	para-Cymene
9.80%	-	Limonene
3.00%	-	Sabinene
2.70%	-	6-Methyl-5-hepten-2-one
2.60%	-	alpha-Pinene
2.60%	-	Methoxy-cymene
1.80%	-	ar-Curcumene
1.50%	-	beta-Pinene
1.50%	-	beta-Selinene
1.50%	-	Germacrene D
1.50%	-	gamma-Curcumene
1.30%	-	alpha-Phellandrene
1.30%	-	beta-Caryophyllene
1.00%	-	beta-Farnesene

0.70%	-	(E)-beta-Ocimene	
0.70%	-	cis-Sabinene hydrate	
0.60%	-	(Z)-beta-Ocimene	
0.50%	-	Terpinolene	
0.50%	-	alpha-Humulene	
0.50%	-	beta-Elemene	
0.50%	-	beta-Cubebene	
0.40%	-	Terpinen-4-ol	
0.30%	-	gamma-Terpinene	
0.30%	-	delta-Cadinene	
0.10%	-	alpha-Thujene	
0.10%	-	trans-Sabinene hydrate	
0.10%	-	Tetradecane	
92.30		TOTAL %	29 COMPOUNDS

Sphaeranthus cyathuloides (Kenya)

BOTANICAL SPECIES

Sphaeranthus cyathuloides O. Hoffm., fam. Asteraceae (Compositae)

AUTHOR

Mwangi, J.W., Achola, K J., Laurent, R., Lwande, W., and Hassanali, A.

TITLE

Essential Oil Constituents of Sphaeranthus cyathuloides O. Hoffm.

PUBLICATION

J. Essent. Oil Res., Vol. 7, 177-178 (Mar/Apr 1995)

COMPOUNDS

67.43%	-	trans-Dihydrocarvone	
26.16%	-	cis-Dihydrocarvone	
1.47%	-	Isodihydrocarveol	
1.34%	-	Neoisodihydrocarveol	
0.44%	-	Limonene	
0.10%	-	Carvone	
0.10%	-	alpha-Humulene	
0.10%	-	beta-Selinene	
0.10%	-	Eugenol	
0.10%	-	alpha-Guaiene	
97.34		TOTAL %	10 COMPOUNDS

Sphaeranthus suaveolens (Egypt)

BOTANICAL SPECIES

Sphaeranthus suaveolens DC., fam. Asteraceae (Compositae)

AUTHOR

De Pooter, H.L., De Buyck, L.F., Schamp, N.M., Harraz, F.M. and El-Shami I.M.

TITLE

The Essential Oil of Sphaeranthus suaveolens DC.

PUBLICATION

Fiav. Fragr. J., Vol. 6, 157-159 (1991)

COMPOUNDS

33.50%	-	Isopinocamphone
16.10%	-	Thymohydroquinone dimethylether
10.60%	-	alpha-Pinene
6.60%	-	1, 8-Cineole
6.30%	-	para-Cymene
4.10%	-	alpha-Phellandrene
1.50%	-	Sabinene
1.20%	-	alpha-Terpinyl acetate
1 20%	-	delta-Cadinene
1.10%	-	gamma-Terpinene
1.00%	-	Pinocamphone
0.90%	-	beta-Caryophyllene
0 70%	-	Terpinen-4-ol
0.70%	-	Spathulenol
0.60%	-	Myrcene
0.60%	-	alpha-Terpineol
0.40%	-	p-Cymen-8-ol

0.40%	-	Caryophyllene oxide
0.30%	-	Carvacrol
0.30%	-	l-Octenol-3
0.30%	-	Pinanol
0.20%	-	Thymol
0.10%	-	alpha-Thujene
0.10%	-	Camphene
0.10%	-	beta-Farnesene
0.10%	-	Nerolidol (unknown isomer)
0.10%	-	Methyl thymol
0.01%	-	alpha-Terpinene
0.01%	-	alpha-Humulene
0.01%	-	alpha-Ylangene
0.01%	-	Eugenol
0.01%	-	beta-Elemene
0.01%	-	Cuminaldehyde
0.01%	-	allo-Aromadendrene
89.17		TOTAL % 34 COMPOUNDS

Tagetes argentina 1 (Argentina)

BOTANICAL SPECIES

Tagetes argentina Cabrera, fam. Asteraceae (Compositae)

AUTHOR

Zygadio, J.A., Maestri, D.M. and Espinar, L.A.

TITLE

The Volatile Oil of Tagetes argentina Cabrera (oil of red stemmed plants)

PUBLICATION

J. Essent. Oil Res., Vol. 5, 85-86 (Jan/Feb 1993)

COMPOUNDS

43.62%	-	(Z)-Ocimenone	
40.36%	-	(E)-Ocimenone	
6.57%	-	Dihydrotagetone	
2.00%	-	(E)-beta-Ocimene	
1.87%	-	(E)-Tagetone	
1.77%	-	(Z)-Tagetone	
1.49%	-	(Z)-beta-Ocimene	
1.27%	-	Neryl acetate	
0 59%	-	Linalool	
0.01%	-	alpha-Pinene	
0.01%	-	beta-Pinene	
99.58		TOTAL %	11 COMPOUNDS

Tagetes argentina 2 (Argentina)

BOTANICAL SPECIES

Tagetes argentina Cabrera, fam. Asteraceae (Compositae)

AUTHOR

Zygadlo, J.A., Maestri, D.M. and Espinar, L.A.

TITLE

The Volatile Oil of Tagetes argentina Cabrera (oil of yellow stemmed plants)

PUBLICATION

J. Essent. Oil Res., Vol. 5, 85-86 (Jan/Feb 1993)

COMPOUNDS

45.59%	-	(Z)-Ocimenone	
37.29%	-	(E)-Ocimenone	
7.26%	-	(E)-beta-Ocimene	
3.82%	-	Dihydrotagetone	
1.46%	-	(Z)-beta-Ocimene	
1.30%	-	(E)-Tagetone	
1.29%	-	(Z)-Tagetone	
0.82%	-	Neryl acetate	
0.61%	-	Linalool	
0.01%	-	alpha-Pinene	
0.01%	-	beta-Pinene	
99.46		TOTAL %	11 COMPOUNDS

Tagetes argentina 3 (Argentina)

BOTANICAL SPECIES

Tagetes argentina Cabrera, fam. Asteraceae (Compositae)

AUTHOR

Zydaglo, J.A., A.L. Lamarque, D.M. Meastri, C.A. Guzman & N.R. Grosso

TITLE

Composition of the Inflorescence Oils of Some Tagetes Species from Argentina

PUBLICATION

J. Essent. Oil Res, Vol. 5, 679-681 (Nov/Dec 1993)

COMPOUNDS

44.00%	-	(Z)-Tagetenone	
38.30%	-	(E)-Tagetenone	
4.10%	-	(E)-beta-Ocimene	
2 10%	-	(E)-Tagetone	
2.10%	-	(Z)-Tagetone	
1.50%	-	(Z)-beta-Ocimene	
0.05%	-	aipha-Pinene	
0.05%	-	beta-Pinene	
0.05%	-	Limonene	
0.05%	-	Neryl acetate	
0.05%	-	Hexanal	
0.05%	-	beta-Eudesmol	
0.05%	-	Heptanal	
92.45		TOTAL %	13 COMPOUNDS

Tagetes filifolia (Argentina) 1

BOTANICAL SPECIES

Tagetes filifolia Lag., fam. Asteraceae (Compositae)

AUTHOR

Zygadio, J.A., A.L. Lamarque, D.M. Maestri, C.A. Guzman & N.R. Grosso

TITLE

Composition of the Inflorescence Oils of Some Tagetes Species from Argentina

PUBLICATION

J. Essent. Oil Res., Voi. 5, 679-681 (Nov/Dec 1993)

COMPOUNDS

67.00%	-	(E)-Anethole	
30.30%	-	Methyl chavicol	
1.00%	-	Dihydrotagetone	
0 05%	-	alpha-Pinene	
0.05%	-	Limonene	
0.05%	-	(Z)-beta-Ocimene	
0.05%	-	(E)-beta-Ocimene	
0.05%	-	Anisaldehyde	
0 05%	-	Methyl isoeugenol	
0.05%	-	Eugenyl acetate	
98.65		TOTAL %	10 COMPOUNDS

Tagetes filifolia (Argentina) 2

BOTANICAL SPECIES

Tagetes filifolia Lag., fam. Asteraceae (Compositae)

AUTHOR

Zygadio, J.A., Guzman, C.A. & N.R. Grosso

TITLE

Antifungal Properties of the Leaf Oils of Tagetes minuta L. and T. filifolia Lag. (trace = 0.01%)

PUBLICATION

J. Essent. Oil Res., Vol. 6, 617-621 (Nov/Dec 1994)

COMPOUNDS

71.30%	-	(E)-Anethole	
20.50%	-	Methyl chavicol	
0.90%	-	Methyl eugenol	
0.90%	-	Dihydrotagetone	
0.01%	-	alpha-Pinene	
0.01%	-	Sabinene	
0.01%	-	beta-Pinene	
0.01%	-	Limonene	
0.01%	-	(Z)-beta-Ocimene	
0.01%	-	(E)-beta-Ocimene	
0.01%	-	Anisaldehyde	
0.01%	-	Eugenyl acetate	
93.58		TOTAL %	12 COMPOUNDS

Tagetes laxa (Argentina)

BOTANICAL SPECIES

Tagetes laxa Cabrera, fam. Asteraceae (Compositae)

AUTHOR

Zygadio, J.A., A.L. Lamarque, D.M. Maestri, C.A. Guzman & N.R. Grosso

TITLE

Composition of the Inflorescence Oils of some Tagetes Species from Argentina

PUBLICATION

J. Essent. Oil Res., Vol. 5, 679-681 (Nov/Dec 1993)

COMPOUNDS

33.20%	-	(E)-Tagetenone
27.10%	-	(Z)-Tagetenone
15.80%	-	(Zy-beta-Ocimene
8.70%	-	(E)-beta-Ocimene
6.20%	-	Dihydrotagetone
5.60%	-	(Z)-Tagetone
0.50%	-	beta-Phellandrene
0.05%	-	alpha-Pinene
0.05%	-	beta-Pinene
0.05%	-	Limonene
0.05%	-	Neryl acetate
0.05%	-	Hexanal
0.05%	-	beta-Eudesmol
0.05%	-	Heptanal
0.05%	-	(E)-Tagetone
97.50	TOTAL %	15 COMPOUNDS

Tagetes lemmonii

BOTANICAL SPECIES

Tagetes lemmonii Gray, fam. Asteraceae (Compositae)

AUTHOR

Tucker, A.O., and Maciarello, M.J.

TITLE

Volatile Leaf oil of Tagetes lemmonii Gray

PUBLICATION

J. Essent. Oil Res., Vol. 8, 417-418 (Jul/Aug 1996)

COMPOUNDS

42.52%	-	Dihydrotagetone	
16.10%	-	(E)-Tagetone	
14.18%	-	(E)-Ocimenone	
3.89%	-	(Z)-Ocimenone	
2.78%	-	Alloocimene (unknown isomer)	
2.14%	-	(E)-beta-Ocimene	
0.46%	-	Germacrene D	
0.39%	-	beta-Caryophyllene	
0.33%	-	Ethyl 2-methylbutyrate	
0.06%	-	alpha-Phellandrene	
0.04%	-	(Z)-Tagetone	
82.99		TOTAL %	11 COMPOUNDS

Tagetes lucida (Hungary)

BOTANICAL SPECIES

Tagetes lucida L, fam. Asteraceae (Compositae)

AUTHOR

Hethelyi, E, Danos, B., Tetenyi, P., and Koczka, I.

TITLE

GC/MS Analysis of Essential Oils of some Tagetes Species

PUBLICATION

In: Progress in Essential Oil Research (Proc. Intern. Symp, on Ess. Oils), E.-J. Brunke, Ed., Walter de Gruyter, Berlin (1986), 131-137

COMPOUNDS

28.00%	-	beta-Caryophyllene	
16.50%	-	Limonene	
13.80%	-	(E)-beta-Ocimene	
58 30		TOTAL %	3 COMPOUNDS

Tagetes (Argentina) 1

BOTANICAL SPECIES

Tagetes minuta L. (Marigold), fam. Asteraceae (Compositae)

AUTHOR

Zygadio, J.A., Grosso, N.R., Abbura, R.E., and Guzman, C.

TITLE

Essential oil variation in Tagetes minuta populations (Tagetes oils from plants grown in 5 regions of Argentina)

PUBLICATION

Systemat. Ecol, Vol. 18, 405-407 (1990)

COMPOUNDS

30.00%	-	(Z)-beta-Ocimene	
30.00%	-	(E)-Tagetenone	
20.00%	-	(E)-beta-Ocimene	
9.44%	-	(E)-Tagetone	
3.85%	-	(Z)-Tagetone	
1.55%	-	Eudesmols (unknown isomer)	
1.10%	-	beta-Pinene	
0.66%	-	Geranyl acetate	
0.65%	-	Linalool	
0.62%	-	alpha-Terpineol	
0.55%	-	Neryl acetate	
0.30%	-	alpha-Pinene	
0.16%	-	Sabinene	
98.88		TOTAL %	13 COMPOUNDS

Tagetes (India) 1

BOTANICAL SPECIES

Tagetes minuta L. (Marigold), fam. Asteraceae (Compositae)

AUTHOR

Gupta, Y.N., and Bhandari, K.S.

TITLE

Essential Oil from the Leaves of Tagetes minuta

PUBLICATION

Indian Pert., Vol. 19 (1), 29-32 (1975)

COMPOUNDS

20.00%	-	Myrcene
18.00%	-	Aromadendrene
15.00%	-	(Z)-beta-Ocimene
8.50%	-	Limonene
6.50%	-	Carvone
5.00%	-	Linalool oxides (cis/trans) (unknown isomers)
3.50%	-	Linalool
2.50%	-	1, 8-Cineole
2.50%	-	Linalyl acetate
2.50%	-	Salicylaldehyde
84.00	TOTAL %	10 COMPOUNDS

Tagetes (India) 2

BOTANICAL SPECIES

Tagetes minuta L. (Marigold), fam. Asteraceae (Compositae)

AUTHOR

Baslas, R.K., and Singh, A.K.

TITLE

Chemical Examination of Essential Oil of Tagetes minuta L.

PUBLICATION

J. Indian Chem. Soc., Vol. 28, 422-423 (1981)

COMPOUNDS

23.90%	-	Aromadendrene	
16.40%	-	Myrcene	
15.10%	-	(E)-Tagetone	
13 10%	-	(Z)-beta-Ocimene	
9.60%	-	Limonene	
6.10%	-	Carvone	
4.30%	-	Linalyl acetate	
3.60%	-	Linalool	
1 04%	-	beta-Phellandrene	
0.96%	-	alpha-Pinene	
0.47%	-	Eugenol	
0.43%	-	para-Cymene	
0.36%	-	beta-Caryophyllene	
95.36		TOTAL %	13 COMPOUNDS

Tagetes (USA) 1

BOTANICAL SPECIES

Tagetes minuta L. (Marigoid), fam. Asteraceae (Compositae)

AUTHOR

Lawrence, B.M.

TITLE

Essential Oils of the Tagetes Genus (North American produced oils)

PUBLICATION

Pert. Flav., Vol. 10, Oct./Nov. 1985, 73-82

COMPOUNDS

40.00%	-	(Z)-beta-Ocimene
15.80%	-	(Z)-Tagetenone
15.15%	-	Dihydcotagetolen-2-one
11.50%	-	(Z)-Tagetone
5.50%	-	(E)-Tagetenone
0.05%	-	Limonene
88.00	TOTAL %	6 COMPOUNDS

Tagetes 1

BOTANICAL SPECIES

Tagetes minuta L. (Marigold), fam. Asteraceae (Compositae)

AUTHOR

Lawrence, B.M.

TITLE

Essential Oils of the Tagetes Genus (5 commercial samples)

PUBLICATION

Perf. Flav., Vol. 10, Oct./Nov. 1985, 73-82

COMPOUNDS

42.30%	-	(Z)-beta-Ocimene	
11.40%	-	Dihydrotagetolen-2-one	
6.00%	-	Limonene	
4.70%	-	(Z)-Tagetone	
2.50%	-	(Z)-Tagetenone	
1.00%	-	(E)-Tagetenone	
67.90		TOTAL %	6 COMPOUNDS

Tagetes 2

BOTANICAL SPECIES

Tagetes minuta L. (Marigold), fam. Asteraceae (Compositae)

AUTHOR

Lawrence, B.M., Powell, R.H., Smith, T.W., and Kramer, S.W.

TITLE

Chemical composition of Tagetes oil

PUBLICATION

Pert. Flav., Vol. 10 (6), 56-58, (1985-1986)

COMPOUNDS

40.42%	-	(Z)-beta-Ocimene
17.64%	-	Diriydrolagetone
13.00%	-	(Z)-Tagetenone
9.96%	-	(Z)-Tagetone
5.30%	-	(E)-Tagetenone
1.07%	-	(E)-Tagetone
0.87%	-	Thymohydroquinone dimethylether
0.77%	-	gamma-Elemene
0.52%	-	(E)-beta-Ocimene
0.52%	-	beta-Caryophyllene
0.50%	-	beta-Thujone
0.50%	-	Germacrene D
0.50%	-	Methyl thymol
0.41%	-	Linalool
0.41%	-	cis-Alloocimene
0.35%	-	alpha-Phellandrene
0.30%	-	Myrcene
0.29%	-	Linalyl acetate

0.29% - alpha-Humulene
0.27% - Menthol
0.25% - beta-Elemene
0.20% - Ethyl 2-methylbutyrate
0.19% - Methyl chavicol
0.19% - cis-Ocimene epoxide
0.16% - Thymol
0.10% - Geraniol
0.10% - Carvone
0.10% - alpha, p-Dimethylstyrene
0.08% - Isoamyl acetate
0.07% - beta-Phellandree
0.06% - para-Cymene
0.05% - alpha-Thujene
0.05% - (E)-beta-Farnesene
0.05% - Isoplperitenone
0.05% - Naphthalene
0.04% - Piperitenone
0.03% - alpha-Pinene
0.03% - Campnene
0.03% - beta-Pinene
0.03% - Limonene
0.03% - Methyl eugenol
0.03% - (E)-Nerolidol
0.03% - trans-Alloocimene
0.03% - Acetone
0.02% - delta-Cadinene
0.02% - alpha-Cadinol
0.02% - Acetaldehyde
0.02% - Methyl carvacrol
0.02% - Toluene

0.01%	-	Sabinene	
0.01%	-	gamma-Terpinene	
0.01%	-	Terpinolene	
0.01%	-	Borneol	
0.01%	-	Terpinen-4-ol	
0.01%	-	alpha-Terpineol	
0.01%	-	alpha-Thujone	
0.01%	-	Eugenol	
0.01%	-	Carvacrol	
0.01%	-	trans-beta-Bergamotene	
0.01%	-	beta-Eudesmol	
0.01%	-	2-Phenylethanol	
96.09		TOTAL %	61 COMPOUNDS

Tagetes (India) 5

BOTANICAL SPECIES

Tagetes minuta L. (Marigold), fam. Asteraceae (Compositae)

AUTHOR

Thappa, R.K., S,G. Agarwal, N K. Kalia & R. Kapoor

TITLE

Changes in Chemical Composition of Tagetes minuta Oil at Various Stages of Flowering and Fruiting (flower buds, oil yield 0.33%)

PUBLICATION

J. Essent. Oil Res., Vol. 5(4), 375-379 (Jul/Aug 1993)

COMPOUNDS

48.09%	-	Dihydrotagetone	
27.15%	-	(Z)-Tagetone	
16.63%	-	(Z)-beta-Ocimene	
4.60%	-	(Z)-Tagetenone	
3.50%	-	(E)-Tagetenone	
99.97		TOTAL%	5 COMPOUNDS

Tagetes (India) 4

BOTANICAL SPECIES

Tagetes minuta L. (Marigold), fam. Asteraceae (Compositae)

AUTHOR

Thappa, R.K., S.G. Agarwal, N.K. Kalia & R. Kapoor

TITLE

Changes in Chemical Composition of Tagetes minuta Oil at Various Stages of Flowering and Fruiting (mature fruit, yield 1.25%)

PUBLICATION

J. Essent. Oil Res., Vol. 5(4), 375-379 (Jul/Aug 1993)

COMPOUNDS

21.08%	-	(Z)-Tagetone
18.22%	-	(Z)-beta-Ocimene
15.00%	-	(E)-Tagetenone
12.52%	-	(Z)-Tagetenone
11.90%	-	Dihydrotagetone
5.03%	-	(E)-tagetone
83.85	TOTAL %	6 COMPOUNDS

Tagetes (Argentina) 2a

BOTANICAL SPECIES

Tagetes minuta L. (Marigold), fam. Asteraceae (Compositae)

AUTHOR

Zydaglo, J.A., C.A. Guzman & N.R. Grosso

TITLE

Antifungal Properties of the Leaf Oils of Tagetes minuta L. and T. filifolia Lag. (sample from Copina, Argentina) (0.01% = trace)

PUBLICATION

J. Essent. Oil Res., Vol. 6, 617-621 (Nov/Dec) 1994

COMPOUNDS

35.60%	-	(E)-Ocimenone	
32.10%	-	(Z)-Ocimenone	
20.00%	-	(Z)-beta-Ocimene	
6.00%	-	(E)-Tagetone	
2.00%	-	(Z)-Tagetone	
1.00%	-	beta-Eudesmol	
0.70%	-	(E)-beta-Ocimene	
0.01%	-	alpha-Pinene	
0.01%	-	Sabinene	
0.01%	-	beta-Pinene	
0.01%	-	Limonene	
0.01%	-	beta-Phellandrene	
0.01%	-	Neryl acetate	
0.01%	-	Hexanal	
0.01%	-	Heptanal	
0.01%	-	Eugenyl acetate	
0.01%	-	Dihydrotagetone	
97.50		TOTAL %	17 COMPOUNDS

Tagetes (Argentina) 2b

BOTANICAL SPECIES

Tagetes minuta L. (Marigold), fam. Asteraceae (Compositae)

AUTHOR

Zygadlo, J.A., C.A. Guzman & N.R. Grosso

TITLE

Anti fungal Properties of the Leaf Oils of Tagetes minuta L. and T. filifolia Lag. (sample from S. Curvas, Argentina) (0.01% = trace)

PUBLICATION

J. Essent. Oil Res., Vol. 6, 617-621 (Nov/Dec 1994)

COMPOUNDS

40.20%	-	(E)-beta-Ocimene
35.40%	-	(Z)-beta-Ocimene
12.30%	-	(E)-Tagetone
3.20%	-	(Z)-Tagetone
2.00%	-	beta-Pinene
2.00%	-	(Z)-Ocimenone
0.90%	-	(E)-Ocimenone
0.01%	-	alpha-Pinene
0.01%	-	Sabinene
0.01%	-	alpha-Phellandrene
0.01%	-	Limonene
0.01%	-	Neryl acetate
0.01%	-	Hexanal
0.01%	-	10-epi-gamma-Eudesmol
0.01%	-	Heptanal
0.01%	-	Eugenyl acetate
0.01%	-	Dihydrotagetone
96.10	TOTAL%	17 COMPOUNDS

Tagetes (India) 3

BOTANICAL SPECIES

Tagetes minuta L. (Marigold), fam. Asteraceae (Compositae)

AUTHOR

Singh, B., Sood, R.P., and Singh V.

TITLE

Chemical composition of Tagetes minuta L. oil from Himachal Pradesh (India)

PUBLICATION

J. Essent. Oil Res., Vol. 4, 525-526 (1992)

COMPOUNDS

39.44%	-	(Z)-beta-Ocimene
15.43%	-	Dihydrotagetone
14.83%	-	(E)-Ocimenone
9 15%	-	(Z)-Ocimenone
8.78%	-	(Z)-Tagetone
1.89%	-	2, 3, 5-Trimethylfuran
1.65%	-	Isopropyl butyrate
0.92%	-	2-Isobutylnorbonane
0.77%	-	Carvone
0.69%	-	Elemene (unknown isomer)
0.62%	-	Octanal
0.58%	-	beta-Caryophyllene
0.49%	-	(E)-Tagetone
0.41%	-	Piperitone
0.36%	-	Thymol
0.33%	-	Isopropyl propionate
0.28%	-	Decenal (unknown isomer)
0.26%	-	1-Octanol
0.23%	-	2-Methylbutyl acetate
0.22%	-	Sabinene
97.33	TOTAL%	20 COMPOUNDS

Tagetes (USA) 2

BOTANICAL SPECIES

Tagetes minuta L. (Marigold), fam. Asteraceae (Compositae)

AUTHOR

Wells, C., Bertsch, W., and Perich, M.

TITLE

Insecticidal volatiles from the marigold plant (Genus Tagetes). Effect of species and sample manipulations

PUBLICATION

Chromatographia, Vol. 35, 209-215 (1993)

COMPOUNDS

54.57%	-	Tagetone
28.35%	-	(Z)-beta-Ocimene
4.40%	-	Dihydrotagetone
1.76%	-	Limonene
1.12%	-	Germacrene B
1.03%	-	Alloocimene (unknown isomer)
0.52%	-	beta-Caryophyllene
0.50%	-	(E)-Tagetenone
0.40%	-	alpha-Humulene
0.40%	-	cis-Limonene-1, 2-epoxide
0.36%	-	2,2′, 5′, 2″-Terthiopnene
0.33%	-	(E)-beta-Ocimene.
0.20%	-	5-Methyl-2,2′, 5′,2″-terthiophene
0.19%	-	Germacrene D
0.19%	-	1-Octanol
0.18%	-	Sabinene
0.17%	-	alpha-Phellandrene

0.15%	-	5-(But-3-en-1-ynyl)-2,2′-bithiopnene
0.13%	-	(Z)-Tagetenone
0.12%	-	Globulol
0.08%	-	1-Decanol
0.08%	-	Decyl acetate
0.07%	-	Myrcene
0.07%	-	delta-Elemene
0.05%	-	Terpinen-4-ol
0.05%	-	Viridiflorol
0.04%	-	1, 3, 8-p-Menthatriene
0.03%	-	5-(But-3-en-2-ynyl) 5′-methyl-2, 2′ bithiophene
0.03%	-	5-(4-Acetoxy-1-butynyl)-2,2′-bithiophene
0.02%	-	delta-Cadinene
0.01%	-	alpha-Pinene
0.01%	-	para-Cymene
0.01%	-	gamma-Terpinene
0.01%	-	Spathulenol
95.63		TOTAL % 34 COMPOUNDS

Tagetes 3a (leaf)

BOTANICAL SPECIES

Tagetes minuta L. (Marigold), fam. Asteraceae (Compositae)

AUTHOR

Weaver, O.K., et al.

TITLE

Insecticidal activity of floral, foliar and root extracts of Tagetes minuta (Asterales: Asteraceae) against adult Mexican bean weavils (Coleoptea:B)

PUBLICATION

J. Econ. Entomol., Vol. 87, 1718-1725 (1994)

COMPOUNDS

47.50%	-	Dihydrotagetone
9.60%	-	Limonene
6.00%	-	(E)-Tagetone
4.60%	-	(Z)-Tagetone
2.60%	-	(Z)-beta-Ocimene
2.30%	-	5-Methyl-2,2′, 5′,2″-terthiophene
1.50%	-	alpha-Humulene
1.10%	-	Linalool
0.80%	-	Germacrene B
0.40%	-	2,2′, 5′,2″-Terthiophene
0.20%	-	para-Cymene
0.15%	-	Alloocimene (unknown isomer)
0.15%	-	cis-Ocimene epoxide
0.10%	-	Germacrene D
77.00	TOTAL %	14 COMPOUNDS

Tagetes 3b (flower)

BOTANICAL SPECIES

Tagetes minuta L. (Marigold), fam. Asteraceae (Compositae)

AUTHOR

Weaver, D.K., et al.

TITLE

Insecticidal activity of floral, foliar and root extracts of Tagetes minuta (Asterales: Asteraceae) against adult Mexican bean weavils (Coleoptea:B)

PUBLICATION

J. Econ. Entomol., Vol. 87, 1718-1725 (1994)

COMPOUNDS

31.90%	-	(Z)-beta-Ocimene
19.10%	-	(E)-Tagetone
13.50%	-	Dihydrotagetone
5.60%	-	(Z)-Tagetone
3.80%	-	Limonene
2.10%	-	Germacrene B
2.10%	-	2,2′, 5′,2″-Terthiophene
2.00%	-	alpha-Humulene
1.30%	-	(E)-beta-Ocimene
1.00%	-	5-Methyl-2,2′, 5′,2″-terthiophene
0.80%	-	Alloocimene (unknown isomer)
0.40%	-	Terpinen-4-ol
0.40%	-	cis-Ocimene epoxide
0.10%	-	para-Cymene
0.10%	-	Germacrene D
84.20	TOTAL %	15 COMPOUNDS

Tagetes (Rwanda)

BOTANICAL SPECIES

Tagetes minuta L. (Marigold), fam. Asteraceae (Compositae)

AUTHOR

Chalchat, E.G., Carry, R.-P., and Muhayimana, A.

TITLE

Essential Oil of Tagetes minuta from Rwanda and France: Chemical Composition According to Harvesting Location, Growth Stage and Part of Plant Extr.

PUBLICATION

J. Essent. Oil Res., Vol. 7, 375-386 (1995)

COMPOUNDS

38.00%	-	(Z)-beta-Ocimene
25.00%	-	(Z)-Tagetone
10.00%	-	(Z)-Tagetenone
5.00%	-	(E)-Tagetenone
3.00%	-	Dihydrotagetone
2.50%	-	(E)-Tagetone
1.80%	-	Limonene
1.00%	-	Propyl butyrate
0.50%	-	Isobornyl acetate
0.50%	-	4-Methyl-2-pentanone
0.50%	-	p-Menth-4-en-2-one
0.40%	-	Linalool
0.40%	-	(Z)-3-Hexenol
0 30%	-	Sabinene
0.30%	-	Terpinen-4-ol
0.30%	-	Ethyl 2-methylbutyrate

0.20%	-	para-Cymene
0 20%	-	gamma-Terpinene
0.20%	-	cis-Ocimene epoxide
0.20%	-	3, 4-Dimethyloct-2, 4, 6-triene
0.10%	-	Santene
0.10%	-	Myrcene
0.10%	-	alpha-Phellandrene
0.10%	-	delta-3-Carene
0.10%	-	(E)-beta-Ocimene
0.10%	-	1.8-Cineole
0.10%	-	Bornyl acetate
0.10%	-	Artemisia ketone
0.10%	-	2-Hexenal
0.10%	-	Acetone
0.10%	-	Ethyl pentanoate
0.10%	-	2(10)-Pinen-4-one
0.05%	-	alpha-Pinene
0.05%	-	Camphene
0.05%	-	beta-Pinene
91.65		TOTAL % 35 COMPOUNDS

Tagetes (France)

BOTANICAL SPECIES

Tagetes minuta L. (Marigold), fam. Asteraceae (Compositae)

AUTHOR

Chalchat, J.-C., Garry, R.-P., and Muhayimana, A.

TITLE

Essential Oil of Tagetes minuta from Rwanda and France: Chemical Composition According to Harvesting Location, Growth Stage and Part of Plant Extr.

PUBLICATION

J. Essent. Oil Res., Vol. 7, 375-386 (Jul/Aug 1995); (analysis of oil of whole plant)

COMPOUNDS

40.00%	-	(Z)-beta-Ocimene
33.40%	-	(Z)-Tagetenone
3.70%	-	(E)-Tagetenone
3.20%	-	Limonene
3.00%	-	(Z)-Tagetone
1.90%	-	Isobornyl acetate
1.60%	-	Terpinen-4-ol
1.50%	-	Dinydrotagetone
1.10%	-	p-Menth-4-en-2-one
0.70%	-	(E)-Tagetone
0.60%	-	3, 4-Dimethyloct-2, 4, 6-triene
0.40%	-	Sabinene
0.40%	-	gamma-Terpinene
0.30%	-	alpha-Phellandrene
0.30%	-	2(10)-Pinen-4-one
0.20%	-	cis-Ocimene epoxide

0.10%	-	alpha-Pinene
0.10%	-	Myrcene
0.10%	-	para-Cymene
0.10%	-	Artemisia ketone
0.10%	-	Ethyl 2-metnylbutyrate
0.10%	-	Ethyl pentanoate
0.05%	-	Santene
0.05%	-	alpha-Thujene
0.05%	-	Camphene
0.05%	-	beta-Pinene
0.05%	-	delta-3-Carene
0.05%	-	Linalool
0.05%	-	1, 8-Cineole
0.05%	-	Bornyl acetate
0.05%	-	(Z)-3-Hexenol
0.05%	-	2-Hexenal
0.05%	-	Acetone
0.05%	-	4-Methyl-2-pentanone
0.05%	-	Propyl butyrate
93.55		TOTAL% 35 COMPOUNDS

Tagetes minuta (Hungary)

BOTANICAL SPECIES

Tagetes minuta L. (T.glandulifera Schrank), fam. Asteraceae (Compositae)

AUTHOR

Hethelyi, E., Danos, B., Tetenyi, P., and Koczka, I.

TITLE

GC/MS Analysis of Essential Oils of some Tagetes Species

PUBLICATION

In : Progress in Essential Oil Research (Proc. Intern. Symp. on Ess. Oils), E.J. Brunke, Ed., Walter de Gruyter, Berlin (1986), 131-137

COMPOUNDS

38.60%	-	(E)-beta-Ocimene	
26.00%	-	(E)-Ocimenone	
10.70%	-	(E) Tagetone	
10.60%	-	Dihydrotagetolen-2-one	
5.00%	-	(Z)-Ocimenone	
90.90		TOTAL %	5 COMPOUNDS

Tagetes (Turkey)

BOTANICAL SPECIES

Tagetes minuta L. (T. glandulifera Schrank), fam. Asteraceae (Compositae)

AUTHOR

Baser, K.H.C., and Maiyer, H.

TITLE

Essential Oil of Tagetes minuta L. from Turkey

PUBLICATION

J. Essent. Oil Res., vol. 8, 337-338 (May/Jun 1996)

COMPOUNDS

30.30% - Dihydrotagetone
28.49% - (Z)-beta-Ocimene
15.35% - (E)-Tagetenone
7 24% - Limonene
4.80% - (E)-Tagetone
1.87% - (Z)-Tagetenone
0.96% - Sabinene
0 47% - beta-Caryophyllene
0.39% - (E)-beta-Ocimene
0.32% - Alloocimene (unknown isomer)
0.26% - Isopiperitenone
0.25% - (Z)-Tagetone
0 12% - Decanal
0.10% - Myrcene
0.10% - Bicyciogermacrene
0.09% - alpha-Phellandrene
0 08% - Ethyl 2-methylbutyrate

0.07%	-	beta-Phellandrene	
0.06%	-	alpha-Pinene	
0.06%	-	(E)-2-Hexenal	
0.05%	-	gamma-Terpinene	
0.02%	-	alpha-Terpinene	
91.45		TOTAL %	22 COMPOUNDS

Tagetes patula (Hungary)

BOTANICAL SPECIES

Tagetes patula L., fam. Asteraceae (Compositae)

AUTHOR

Hethelyi, E., Danos, B., Tettenyi, P., and Kockzka, I.

TITLE

GC/MS Analysis of Essential Oils of some Tagetes Species

PUBLICATION

In: Progress in Essential Oil Research (Proc. Intern. Symp. on Ess. Oils),E.-J. Brunke, Ed., Walter de Gruyter, Berlin (1986), 131-137

COMPOUNDS

14.20%	-	Limonene	
13.40%	-	(Z)-Ocimenone	
13.40%	-	(E)-Ocimenone	
11.90%	-	beta-Caryophyllene	
11.70%	-	(E)-beta-Ocimene	
7.00%	-	(E)-Tagetone	
3.40%	-	Nerol	
75.00		TOTAL %	7 COMPOUNDS

Tagetes riojana (Argentina)

BOTANICAL SPECIES

Tagetes riojana Ferraro, fam. Asteraceae (Compositae)

AUTHOR

Zygadio, J.A.

TITLE

Volatile Oil of Tagetes riojana Ferraro

PUBLICATION

J. Essent. Oil Res., Vol. 7, 319-320 (May/Jun 1955)

COMPOUNDS

40.29%	-	(E)-Tagetone	
23.18%	-	(Z)-Ocimenone	
15.44%	-	Dihydrotagetone	
7.50%	-	(E)-beta-Ocimene	
4.58%	-	(E)-Ocimenone	
4.49%	-	(Z)-Tagetone	
1.20%	-	(Z)-beta-Ocimene	
0.51%	-	alpha-Pinene	
0.01%	-	beta-Pinene	
0.01%	-	Linalool	
0.01%	-	Neryl acetale	
97.22		TOTAL %	11 COMPOUNDS

Tagetes tenuifolia (Hungary)

BOTANICAL SPECIES

Tagetes tenuifolia Cav. (T.Signata Bartl.), fam. Asteraceae (Compositae)

AUTHOR

Hethelyi, E., Danos, B., Tetenyi, P., and Koczka, I.

TITLE

GC/MS Analysis of Essential Oils of some Tagetes Species

PUBLICATION

In: Progress in Essential Oil Research (Proc. Intern. Symp. on Ess. Oils),E.-J. Brunke, Ed., Walter de Gruyter, Berlin (1986), 131-137

COMPOUNDS

33.80%	-	(E)-Ocimenone	
25.40%	-	(E)-Tagetone	
16.80%	-	Dihydrotagetolen-2-one	
8.30%	-	(E)-beta-Ocimene	
2.70%	-	beta-Caryophyllene	
2.20%	-	(Z)-Ocimenone	
89.20%		TOTAL %	6 COMPOUNDS

Tagetes terniflora (Argentina)

BOTANICAL SPECIES

Tagetes terniflora H.B.K., fam. Asteraceae (Compositae)

AUTHOR

Zygadlo, J.A., A.L. Lamarque, D.M. Maestri, C.A. Guzman & N.R. Grosso

TITLE

Composition of the Inflorescence Oils of Some Tagetes Species from Argentina

PUBLICATION

J. Essent. Oil Res., Vol. 5, 679-681 (Nov/Dec 1993)

COMPOUNDS

68.20%	-	(Z)-Tagetone
15.00%	-	(Z)-beta-Ocimene
5.50%	-	(E)-Tagetenone
3 20%	-	Dihydrotagetone
3.10%	-	(Z)-Tagetenone
1.20%	-	beta-Phellandrene
0.90%	-	(E)-beta-Ocimene
0.05%	-	alpha-Pinene
0.05%	-	beta-Pinene
0.05%	-	Limonene
0.05%	-	Neryl acetate
0.05%	-	Hexanal
0.05%	-	beta-Eudesmol
0.05%	-	Heptanal
0.05%	-	(E)-Tagetone
97.50	TOTAL%	15 COMPOUNDS

Tanacetum parthenium (Belgium)

BOTANICAL SPECIES

Tanacetum parthenium (L.) Schuitz-Bip. (Feverfew), Asteraceae (Compositae)

AUTHOR

Pooter De, H.L., Vermeesch J., and Schamp N.M.

TITLE

The Essential Oils of Tanacetum vulgare L. and Tanacetum parthenium (L.) Schultz-Bip (1 sample Belgium)

PUBLICATION

J. Ess. Oil Res., Vol. 1, no. 1, 9-13 (1989)

COMPOUNDS

44.20%	-	Carvone
23.50%	-	trans-Chrysantenyl acetate
5.40%	-	Camphene
4.60%	-	Germacrene D
3.10%	-	para-Cymene
2.80%	-	Terpinen-4-ol
1.30%	-	Linalool
1 00%	-	alpha-Pinene
1.00%	-	gamma-Terpinene
1.00%	-	Borneol
0.80%	-	beta-Farnesene
0.70%	-	Bornyl acetate
0.60%	-	alpha-Thujene
0.60%	-	alpha-Phellandrene
0.50%	-	Limonene
0.50%	-	Sesquiterpenes, oxygen-containing-

0.05%	-	Sabinene	
0.05%	-	beta-Pinene	
0.05%	-	beta-Caryophyllene	
0.05%	-	delta-Cadinene	
0.05%	-	Pinocarvone	
0.05%	-	Eugenol	
91.90		TOTAL%	22 COMPOUNDS

Tanacetum parthenium (The Netherlands)

BOTANICAL SPECIES

Tanacetum parthenium (L.) Schultz-Bip. (Feverfew), Asteraceae (Compositae)

AUTHOR

Hendriks, H., Bos, R., and Woerdenbag, H.J.

TITLE

The Essential Oii of Tanacetum parthenium (L.) Schuitz-Bip. (analysis of oil of freshly grown sample) (0.01% = trace)

PUBLICATION

Flavour Fragr. J., Vol. 11, 367-371 (1996)

COMPOUNDS

42.73%	-	Camphor
24.00%	-	Chrysanthenyl acetate
6.46%	-	Camphene
3.03%	-	Germacrene D
2.98%	-	alpha-Terpinene
2.52%	-	beta-Farnesene
2.06%	-	Caryophyllene oxide
1.90%	-	Bornyl acetate
1.87%	-	gamma-Terpinene
1.65%	-	alpha-Pinene
1.42%	-	trans-Chrysanthenol
0.70%	-	alpha-Thujene
0.63%	-	para-Cymene
0.60%	-	Borneol
0.53%	-	beta-Caryophyllene
0.33%	-	Sabinene

0.27%	-	beta-Pinene
0.27%	-	Terpinen-4-ol
0.17%	-	alpha-Terpineol
0.14%	-	Pinocarvone
0.10%	-	Sabinene hydrate
0.10%	-	Thujopsene
0.01%	-	Limonene
0.01%	-	Terpinolene
0.01%	-	1, 8-Cineole
0.01%	-	alpha-Humulene
0.01%	-	delta-Cadinene
0.01%	-	alpha-Copaene
0.01%	-	Benzaldehyde
0.01%	-	Thymol
0.01%	-	Carvacrol
0.01%	-	Cuminaldehyde
0.01%	-	Chrysanthenyl angelate
0.01%	-	Linalyl propionate
0.01%	-	alpha, p-Dimethylstyrene
0.01%	-	Curcumene (unknown isomer)
0.01%	-	Benzyl isobutyrate
0.01%	-	Benzyl isovalerate
0.01%	-	4-Ethylbenzaldehyde
0.01%	-	4-Methylbenzaldehyde
0.01%	-	Benzyl propionate
0.01%	-	Chrysanthenyl propionate
0.01%	-	Chrysanthenyl isovalerate
94.67	TOTAL %	43 COMPOUNDS

Tansy (Belgium)

BOTANICAL SPECIES

Tanacetum vulgare L., fam. Asteraceae (Compositae)

AUTHOR

Pooter De, H.L., Vermeesch J., and Schamp N.M.

TITLE

The Essential Oils of Tanacetum vulgare L. and Tanacetum parthenium (L.) Schultz-Bip (4 samples T. vulgare)

PUBLICATION

J. Ess. Oil Res., Vol. 1, no. 1, 9-13 (1989)

COMPOUNDS

50.00%	-	beta-Thujone
20.00%	-	trans-Chrysanlenyl acetate
6.40%	-	Camphor
5.00%	-	Germacrene D
1.80%	-	alpha-Thujone
1.00%	-	Sabinene
0.60%	-	Camphene
0.55%	-	alpha-Pinene
0.55%	-	1, 8-Cineole
0.40%	-	Eugenol
0.30%	-	para-Cymene
0.30%	-	gamma-Terpinene
0.30%	-	Pinocarvone
0.25%	-	Terpinen-4-ol
0.25%	-	beta-Caryophyllene
0.15%	-	beta-Pinene
0.15%	-	Limonene

0.15%	-	Terpinolene	
0.15%	-	delta-Cadinene	
0.15%	-	alpha-Copaene	
0.10%	-	alpha-Terpinene	
0.10%	-	Bornyl acetate	
0.10%	-	Myrtenal	
0.05%	-	trans-Pinocarveol	
0.01%	-	Myrcene	
0.01%	-	alpha-Terpineol	
0.01%	-	Myrtenol	
88.83		TOTAL %	27 COMPOUNDS

Tansy flowers (Canada)

BOTANICAL SPECIES

Tanacetum vulgare L, fam. Asteraceae (Compositae)

AUTHOR

Collin, G.J., H. Deslauriers, N. Pageau & M. Gagnon

TITLE

Essential Oil of Tansy (Tanacetum vulgare L.) of Canadian Origin (oil of flowers of Tanacetum vulgare)

PUBLICATION

J. Essent. Oil Res., Vol.5, 629-638 (1993)

COMPOUNDS

21.60%	-	trans-Dihydrocarvone
13.00%	-	Borneol
13.00%	-	1, 8-Cineole
11.60%	-	beta-Thujone
9.10%	-	Camphor
3.90%	-	Chrysanthenone
3.60%	-	cis-Dihydrocarvone
3.50%	-	Bornyl acetate
3.32%	-	Camphene
3.00%	-	Limonene
2.67%	-	Sabinene
1.86%	-	Umbellulone
1.35%	-	alpha-Pinene
1.05%	-	Germacrene D
1.03%	-	Terpinen-4-ol
1.00%	-	beta-Pinene
0.83%	-	Pinocarvone

0.82%	-	Carvone
0.60%	-	Pinocarveol
0.40%	-	Isodihydrocarveol
0.39%	-	alpha-Terpineol
0.38%	-	gamma-Terpinene
0.36%	-	para-Cymene
0.23%	-	alpha-Terpinene
0.22%	-	Linalool
0.21%	-	Tricyclene
0.20%	-	cis-p-Menth-2-en-l-ol
0.16%	-	Chrysanthenyl acetate
0.10%	-	beta-Phellandrene
0.10%	-	Nerol
0.10%	-	alpha-Copaene
0.10%	-	alpha, p-Dimethylstyrene
0.10%	-	trans-p-Menth-2-en-1-ol
99.88		TOTAL% 33 COMPOUNDS

Tansy stems & sheets (Canada)

BOTANICAL SPECIES

Tanacetum vulgare L, fam. Asteraceae (Compositae)

AUTHOR

Collin, G.J., H. Deslauriers, N. Pageau & M. Gagnon

TITLE

Essential Oil of Tansy (Tanacetum vulgare L.) of Canadian Origin (oil of stems & sheets of Tanacetum vulgare)

PUBLICATION

J. Essent. Oil Res, Vol. 5, 629-638 (1993)

COMPOUNDS

22.65%	-	1, 8-Cineole
21.20%	-	trans-Dihydrocarvone
10.70%	-	beta-Thujone
10.30%	-	Borneol
3.85%	-	Bornyl acetate
2.70%	-	Sabinene
2.30%	-	Chrysanthenone
2.20%	-	cis-Dihydrocarvone
2.07%	-	Camphene
1.40%	-	Camphor
1.24%	-	alpha-Pinene
1.15%	-	cis-p-Menth-2-en-l-ol
1.00%	-	Carvone
0.93%	-	Terpinen-4-ol
0.90%	-	trans-p-Menth-2-en-l-ol
0.86%	-	beta-Pinene
0.84%	-	Umbellulone

0.70%	-	Isodihydrocarveol	
0.67%	-	Pinocarveol	
0.65%	-	Myrcene	
0.60%	-	Pinocarvone	
0.42%	-	alpha-Terpineol	
0.37%	-	gamma-Terpinene	
0.22%	-	Chrysanthenyl acetate	
0.20%	-	alpha-Thujone	
0.18%	-	alpha-Terpinene	
0.15%	-	beta-Phellandrene	
0.10%	-	Tricyclene	
0.10%	-	Limonene	
0.10%	-	Terpinolene	
0.05%	-	Linalool	
0.02%	-	alpha-Copaene	
90.61		TOTAL%	32 COMPOUNDS

Tithonia diversifolia

BOTANICAL SPECIES

Tithonia diversifolia (Hemsl.) A. Gray, fam. Asteraceae (Compositae)

AUTHOR

Lamaty, G., et al.

TITLE

Aromatic Plants of Tropical Central Africa, III. Constituents of the Essential Oil of the Leaves of Tithonia diversifolia A. Gray from Cameroon

PUBLICATION

J. Essent. Oil Res., Vol. 3, 399-402 (Nov/Dec 1991)

COMPOUNDS

40.20%	-	(Z)-beta-Ocimene
25.00%	-	alpha-Pinene
13.90%	-	Limonene
5.80%	-	(E)-beta-Ocimene
2.40%	-	beta-Caryophyllene
1.70%	-	gamma-Elemene
1.30%	-	Caryophyllene oxide
1.30%	-	Nerolidol (unknown isomer)
1.20%	-	Sabinene
1.20%	-	beta-Pinene
0.90%	-	Spathulenol
0.30%	-	Linalool
0.20%	-	alpha-Humulene
0.20%	-	Verbenone
0.10%	-	Terpinen-4-ol
0.10%	-	alpha-Terpineol

0.10%	-	Citronellal	
0.10%	-	delta-Cadinene	
0.10%	-	gamma-Cadinene	
0.01%	-	gamma-Terpinene	
96.11		TOTAL%	20 COMPOUNDS

Vanillosmopsis arborea leaf

BOTANICAL SPECIES

Vanillosmopsis arborea Baker, fam. Asteraceae (Compositae)

AUTHOR

Craveiro, A.A., Alencar, J.W., Matos. F.J.A, Sousa, M.P., Machado, M.I.L

TITLE

Volatil Constituents of Leaves, Bark and Wood From Vanillosmopsis arborea Baker

PUBLICATION

J. Ess. Oil Res, Vol. 1, 293-294, (Nov./Dec. 1989)

COMPOUNDS

23.11%	-	beta-Caryophyllene	
14.17%	-	gamina-Muurolene	
10.90%	-	gamma-Elemene	
7.42%	-	alpha-Humulene	
6.90%	-	alpha-Copaene	
3.53%	-	gamma-Cadinene	
2.52%	-	delta-Elemene	
1.74%	-	alpha-Farnesene	
1.04%	-	(-)-alpha-Bisabolol	
0.74%	-	Safrole	
0.55%	-	beta-Bourbonene	
0.48%	-	alpha-Cubebene	
73.10		TOTAL%	12 COMPOUNDS

Vanillosmopsis arborea bark

BOTANICAL SPECIES

Vanillosmopsis arborea Baker, fam. Asteraceae (Compositae)

AUTHOR

Craveiro, A.A., Alencar, J.W., Matos, F.J.A., Sousa,M.P., Machado, M.I.L

TITLE

Volatile Constituents of Leaves, Bark and Wood From Vanillosmopsis arborea Baker [(2=bark oil; 3=wood oil, which contains (-)-alpha-bisabolol (98%)]

PUBLICATION

J. Ess. Oil Res., Vol. 1, 293-294, (Nov./Dec. 1989)

COMPOUNDS

69.46%	-	(-)-alpha-Bisabolol
5.91%	-	Methyl eugenol
4.06%	-	alpha-Cadinol
3.65%	-	Methyl chavicol
2.68%	-	Elemicin
2.04%	-	beta-Maaliene
1.85%	-	beta-Cubebene
1.83%	-	delta-Elemene
1.20%	-	beta-Elemene
1.00%	-	alpha-Bisabolene
0.75%	-	beta-Himachalene
0.60%	-	beta-Caryophyllene
95.03	TOTAL %	12 COMPOUNDS

Vassaoura (Uruguay)

BOTANICAL SPECIES

Baccharis drancunculifolia DC., fam. Asteraceae (Compositae)

AUTHOR

Loayza, 1., G. Collin, M. Gagnon & E. Dellacasa

TITLE

Huiles essentielles de Baccharis latifolia, B. salicifolia de Bolivie et de B. drancunculifolia en provenance de Uruguay

PUBLICATION

Rivista Ital. EPPOS (Numero Speciale), 728-735 (1993)

COMPOUNDS

20.00%	-	beta-Pinene
14.00%	-	Globulol
9.15%	-	Spathulenol
7.20%	-	Bicyclogermacrene
6.10%	-	beta-Caryophyllene
5.90%	-	alpha-Pinene
3.50%	-	Limonene
3.50%	-	1, 8-Cineole
2.62%	-	deita-Cadinene
2.00%	-	Myrcene
1.38%	-	Germacrene D
1.25%	-	Caryophyllene oxide
0.75%	-	Aromadendrene
0.65%	-	Ledol
0.63%	-	Elemol
0.60%	-	alpha-Humulene

0.57%	-	Cubenol	
0.55%	-	alpha-Terpineol	
0.47%	-	Terpinen-4-ol	
0.30%	-	gamma-Terpinene	
0.25%	-	allo-Aromadendrene	
0.20%	-	Linalool	
81.57		TOTAL %	22 COMPOUNDS

Vassoura (Brazil) 1

BOTANICAL SPECIES

Baccharis dracunculifolia DC., fam. Asteraceae (Compositae)

AUTHOR

Motl, O., and Trka, A.

TITLE

Zusammensetzung des brasilianischen Vassoura Oels (aus Baccharis dracunculifolia)

PUBLICATION

Parfum. Kosmet., Vol. 64, 488-491 (1983)

COMPOUNDS

22.00%	-	Nerolidol (unknown isomer)
16.50%	-	alpha-Pinene
6.40%	-	beta-Caryophyllene
6.40%	-	beta-Elemene
6.40%	-	delta-Elemene
6.40%	-	gamma-Elemene
4.50%	-	beta-Pinene
3.40%	-	Myrcene
2.00%	-	Spathulenol
2.00%	-	Methyl citronellate
2.00%	-	Ethyl dihydrocinnamate
1.40%	-	beta-Phellandrene
1.30%	-	delta-3-Carene
1.30%	-	para-Cymene
82.00	TOTAL%	14 COMPOUNDS

Vassoura (Brazil) 2

BOTANICAL SPECIES

Baccharis dracunculifolia DC., fam. Asteraceae (Compositae)

AUTHOR

Queiroga, C.L, A. Fukai & A.J. Marsaioli

TITLE

Composition of the essential oil of Vassoura (0.01% = present)

PUBLICATION

J. Braz. Chem. Soc., Vol 1 (3), 105-109 (1990)

COMPOUNDS

12.29%	-	Nerolidol (unknown isomer)
5.12%	-	Spathulenol
4.91%	-	delta-Cadinene
4.75%	-	beta-Caryophyllene
4.03%	-	beta-Terpineol
3.60%	-	Aromadendrene
3.54%	-	beta-Cubebene
3.19%	-	Globulol
2.25%	-	alpha-Thujene
2.23%	-	allo-Aromadendrene
2.00%	-	Viridiflorol
0.87%	-	alpha-Copaene
0.80%	-	epi-Globulol
0.54%	-	Cadinol (unknown structure)
0.39%	-	alpha-Cubebene
0.27%	-	4beta, 7beta-Aromadendrandiol
0.01%	-	Sabinene
0.01%	-	para-Cymene

0.01%	-	Limonene
0.01%	-	Terpinen-4-ol
0.01%	-	alpha-Terpineol
0.01%	-	Nerol
0.01%	-	Geraniol
0.01%	-	Citronellal
0.01%	-	Geranial
0.01%	-	Linalyl acetate
0.01%	-	alpha-Humulene
0.01%	-	alpha-Muurolene
0.01%	-	beta-Seliene
0.01%	-	gamma-Cadinene
0.01%	-	alpha-Gurjuene
0.01%	-	Calamenene
0.01%	-	Citronellyl formate
0.01%	-	alpha-lonone
0.01%	-	Palustrol
0.01%	-	alpha-Elemene
0.01%	-	Isolongifólene
0.01%	-	Safranal
0.01%	-	p-1-Menthenal-9
0.01%	-	Isolongifolenol
51.02	TOTAL%	40 COMPOUNDS

Vassoura (Brazil) 3

BOTANICAL SPECIES

Baccharis dracunculifolia DC., fam. Asteraceae (Compositae)

AUTHOR

Weyerstahl, P., Christiansen, C., and Marschall, H.

TITLE

Constituents of Brazilian Vassoura Oil

PUBLICATION

Flavour Fragr. J., Vol. 11, 15-23 (1996)

COMPOUNDS

15.00%	-	(E)-Nerolidol
8.40%	-	Limonene
6.20%	-	beta-Caryophyllene
5.90%	-	beta-Pinene
5.60%	-	delta-Cadinene
3.60%	-	Germacrene D
3.60%	-	Ledene
3.50%	-	Spathulenol
3.30%	-	Aromadendrene
3.10%	-	Bicyclogermacrene
2.90%	-	alpha-Pinene
2.10%	-	gamma-Muurolene
1.90%	-	alpha-Humulene
1.60%	-	beta-Elemene
1.60%	-	alpha-Cadinol
1.30%	-	gamma-Cadinene
1.30%	-	Cabreuva oxide B
1.10%	-	allo-Aromadendrene

1.00%	-	Myrcene
1.00%	-	Globulol
1.00%	-	cis-Calamenene
0.90%	-	alpha-Muurolene
0.90%	-	5, 11-Epoxycadin-1(10)-ene
0.70%	-	Ledol
0.70%	-	Propyl 3-phenylpropanoate
0.65%	-	T-Cadinol
0.65%	-	T-Muurolol
0.60%	-	Caryophyllene oxide
0.60%	-	Palustrol
0.60%	-	Pacifigorgiol
0.60%	-	(E, E)-3, 7, 11-Trimethyldodeca-1, 6, 9 trien 3, 11-diol
0.50%	-	alpha-Terpineol
0.50%	-	Methyl eugenol
0.50%	-	Viridiflorol
0.50%	-	beta-Oplopenone
0.50%	-	trans-Calamenene
0.40%	-	Linalool
0.40%	-	delta-Elemene
0.40%	-	10-epi-Junenol
0.40%	-	Junenol
0.40%	-	(E)-4, 8-Dimethylnona-1, 3, 7 -triene
0.40%	-	Cabreuva oxide D
0.40%	-	Isohumbertiole (unknown isomer)
0.40%	-	2-Methylbutyl 3-phenylpropanoate
0.40%	-	3-Methylbutyl 3-phenylpropanoate
0.40%	-	trans-Dracunculifoliol
0.40%	-	Salvia-4(15)-en-1-one
0.30%	-	Cubenol

0.30% - alpha-Calacorene
0.30% - Cabreuva oxide A
0.30% - 10, 11-Epoxycalamenene
0.30% - cis-Dracunculifoliol
0.30% - exo-1, 5-Epoxysalvial-4(15)-ene
0.30% - Maaliol
0.30% - Germacra-4(15), 5, 10(14)-trien-1beta-ol
0.30% - Waitziacuminone
0.20% - Terpinolene
0.20% - Neryl acetate
0.20% - alpha-Copaene
0.20% - gamma Elemene
0.20% - Acetophenone
0.20% - Ethyl decanoate
0.20% - epi-Globulol
0.20% - 2, 2-Dimethyl-6-vinylchromene
0.20% - 1, 6-Epoxyeudesm-4(15)-ene
0.20% - 4-epi-Maaliol
0.20% - (E)-5-Hydroxynerolidol
0.10% - alpha-Thujene
0.10% - Sabinene
0.10% - para-Cymene
0.10% - gamma-Terpinene
0.10% - Geraniol
0.10% - Myrtenal
0.10% - beta-Damascenone
0.10% - Humulene oxide II
0.10% - Isopropyl 3-phenylpropanoate
0.10% - Cabreuva oxide C
0.10% - 10, 11-Epoxycadina-4, 9-diene
0.10% - endo-1, 5-Epoxysalvial-4(15)-ene

0.10%	-	4(15)-Dehydroglobulol
0.10%	-	Opposita-4(14), 11(12)-dien-1beta-ol
0.10%	-	4-Methyl-6-isopropyl-1-tetralone
0.10%	-	(E, E)-Isobicyclogermacra-1(10),4-dien-15-ol
0.10%	-	(Z)-3-Hexenyl 3-phenylpropanoate
0.08%	-	alpha-Terpinene
0.08%	-	Geranyl acetate
0.08%	-	Ethyl 3-phenylpropionate
0.07%	-	beta-Ionone
0.07%	-	(Z)-4, 8-Dimethylnona-1,3,7-triene
0.05%	-	delta-3-Carene
0.05%	-	Theaspirane (unknown isomer)
0.05%	-	(E)-4,8-Dimethylnona-3,7-dien-2-one
0.05%	-	Isobutyl 3-phenylpropanoate
0.05%	-	sec-Butyl 3-phenyipropanoate
0.03%	-	Terpineh-4-ol
0.03%	-	p-Cymen-8-ol
0.03%	-	Myrtenol
0.63%	-	cis-Carveol
0.63%	-	trans-Carveol
0.03%	-	Vitispirane
0.03%	-	Methyl geranate
0.03%	-	Ethyl octanoate
0.03%	-	(Z)-3-Hexenyl tiglate
0.03%	-	Safranal
0.03%	-	4-Methylacetophenone
0.03%	-	beta-Damascone
0.02%	-	Citronellol
0.02%	-	Nerol
0.02%	-	Geranial

0.02%	-	Safrole
0.02%	-	Anethole
0.02%	-	Methyl phenylpropionate
0.01%	-	Neral
0.01%	-	Carvone
0.01%	-	Cuminaldehyde
0.01%	-	Methyl citronellate
0.01%	-	(Z)-4, 8-Dimethylnona-3, 7-dien-2-one
96.56	TOTAL%	117 COMPOUNDS

Wedelia paludosa (Brazil) 1

BOTANICAL SPECIES

Wedelia paludosa DC. (Mal-me-quer), fam. Asteraceae (Compositae)

AUTHOR

Maia, J.G.S., Ramos, L.S., Luz, A.I.R., da Silva M.L, and Zoghbi, M.d. G.B.

TITLE

Uncommon Brazilian Essential Oils of the Labiatae and Compositae

PUBLICATION

In: Flavors and Fragr.: a World Persp., Lawrence, B.M., Mookherjee, B.D., Willis.B.J. (Eds.),Proc. of the 10th Intern. Congress of Ess. Oils, Fragr. & Flavors, Washington, DC, USA,16-20 Nov. 1986, Elsevier, Amsterdam (1988), 177-188

COMPOUNDS

39.11%	-	alpha-Pinene
11.76%	-	alpha-Phefiandrene
9.01%	-	alpha-Curcumene
6.58%	-	beta-Pinene
6.22%	-	beta-Caryophyllene
5.90%	-	Limonene
4.24%	-	Myrcene
2.93%	-	para-Cymene
2.40%	-	gamma-Elemene
2.38%	-	Borneol
2.22%	-	alpha-Humulene
1.05%	-	delta-Elemene
0.95%	-	Camphene

0.68%	-	Carvone	
0.56%	-	delta-Cadinene	
0.52%	-	Camphor	
0.42%	-	beta-Elemene	
0.29%	-	beta-Cubebene	
0.15%	-	Terpinen-4-ol	
0.14%	-	Copaene (unknown isomer)	
97.51		TOTAL%	20 COMPOUNDS

Wedelia paludosa (Brazil) 2

BOTANICAL SPECIES

Wedelia paludosa DC. (Mal-me-quer), fam. Asteraceae (Compositae)

AUTHOR

Craveiro, A.A., et al.

TITLE

Volatile Constituents of Two Wedelia Species

PUBLICATION

J. Essent. Oil Res., Vol. 5, 439-441 (Jul/Aug 1993)

COMPOUNDS

35.90%	-	alpha-Pinene	
21.30%	-	Limonene	
11.80%	-	gamma-Muurolene	
10.30%	-	beta-Pinene	
4.80%	-	alpha-Phellandrene	
3.10%	-	(E)-beta-Ocimene	
2.60%	-	Camphene	
2.30%	-	Myrcene	
2.30%	-	beta-Caryophyllene	
2.20%	-	(Z)-beta-Ocimene	
2.00%	-	gamma-Elemene	
0.01%	-	Terpinen-4-ol	
0.01%	-	Thymol	
0.01%	-	Phenylacetaldehyde	
0.01%	-	1-Hexanol	
0.01%	-	3-Hexenol-1	
0.01%	-	2-Phenylethanol	
98.66		TOTAL%	17 COMPOUNDS

References

Aalbersberg, W.G.L., and Singh, Y. 1991. Essential Oil of Fijian *Ageratum conyzoides* L. from Suva and Nadi. *Flav. Fragr.J.*, Vol.6,117-120.

Achola, K. J., Munenge, R. W. and Mwaura, A.M. 1994. Pharmacological properties of root and aerial part extracts of *Ageratum conyzoides* on isolated ileum and heart. *Fitoterapia,* 65: 4, 322-325; 8 ref.

Alvarez, L., Marquina, S., Villarreal, M.L., Alonso, D., Aranda, E, and Delgado, G. 1996. Bioactive polyacetylenes from *Bidens pilosa. Planta Medica.*, 62: 4, 355-357. 20 ref.

Anonymous 1973, *Journal of Research in Indian medicine, Yoga and Homeopathy,* New Delhi 8(1), 76.

Anonymous 1991.*Materia Medica of Ayurveda Based on Madanapala's Nighantu* by Vaidya Bhagwan Dash. Assisted by K.V. Kanchan Gupta. Jain Publisher (P) Ltd.

Bamba, D., Bessiere, J.M., Marion, C., Pelissier, Y. and Fouraste, I. 1993. Essential Oil of *Eupatorium Odortatum*. *Planta Medica,* 59:2,184 – 185; 10 ref.

Baruah, R N.and Leclereq, P.A. 1993. Characterization of the essential oil from flower heads of *Spilanthes acmella*. *Journal of Essential oil Research* 5: 6, 693-695; 10 ref.

Baruah, R N.and Leclereq, P.A. 1993. Characterization of the essential oil from flower heads of *Spilanthes acmella*. *Journal of Essential oil Research* 5: 6, 693-695; 10 ref.

Bioka, D., Mabika, A., Abena, A.A., Schilcher, H., Phillipson, J.D., and Loew, D 1993. Analgesic effect of a crude extract of *Ageratum conyzoides* in the rat. First World congress on medicinal and aromatic plants for human welfare (WOCMAP), Maastricht, Netherlands, *Acta Horticulture,* No:332, 171 – 176, 12 ref.

Chandra, S. et al. 1996. Essential Oil Composition of *Ageratum houstonianum* Mill. from Jammu Region of India. *J.Essent Oil Res.,* Vol. 8, 129-134.(March/April).

Craveiro, A.A. et al. 1993. Volatile Constituents of Two *Wedelia* Species. *J. Essent. Oil res.,* Vol. 5, 439-441., (Jul/Aug).

Dung, N.X., Tho, P.T.T., Dan, N.V. and Leclercq, P.A. 1989. Chemical Composition of the Oil of *Ageratum conyzodes* L. from Vietnam. *J. Ess. Oil Res.,* Vol. 1, 135-136. (May/June).

George and Pandalai. 1949. *Indian Journal of Medicinal Research.* Calcutta, 37,169.

Hethelyi, E., Danos, B., Tettenyi, P. and Kockzka, I. 1986. GC/MS Analysis of Essential Oils of some Tagetes Species. In: *Progress in Essential Oil Research* (Proc. Intern. Symp. on Ess. Oils), by E.J. Brunke, (ed.), Walter de Gruyter, Berlin. 131-137.

Johri, R.K. and Singh, C. 1997. Medicinal uses of *Vernonia* species. *Journal of Medicinal and Aromatic Plant Science.* 19:3 744 – 752; 99 ref. L. from Suva and Nadi. *Flav. Fragr.J.,* Vol. 6,117-120.

Lemonica, I.P., and Alvarenga, C.M.D. 1994. Abortive and teratogenic effect of *Acanthospermum hispidum* DC and *Cajanus cajan* (L.) Millps. in pregnant rats. *Journal of Ethnopharmacology.,* 43: 1, 39-44; 16 ref.

Lemos, T.L.G., Pessoa, O.D.L., Matos, F.J.A., Alencar, J.W. and Craveiro, A.A. 1991. The Essential oil of *Spilanthes acmella* Murr. *J. Ess. Oil Res.,* Vol. 3, 369-370. (Sept/Oct).

Machado, M.I.L .et al. 1994. The Presence of Indole as Minor Constituent of *Tagetes erecta* Leaf Oil. *J.Essent. Oil Res.,* Vol. 6, 203-205.(March/April).

Mensah, M., Sarpong, K., Baser, K.H.C. and Ozek, T. 1993. The Essential Oil of *Ageratum conyzoides* L. from Ghana. *J.Essent. Oil Res.*, Vol. 5, 113-115.

Myint, W. 1995. Antihepatotoxic substances from *Eclipta alba* (L) Hassk. (Kyeikhman) *Myanmar – Health Sciences Research Journal* ; 7: 1,9-13 5 ref.

Nadkarni, K.M., 1976. The Indian Materia Medica , 3 rd ed., Popular Prakashan Pvt. Ltd, Bombay, India.

Pattnaik,.S., Subramanyam, V.R. and Kole C. 1996. Anti bacterial and anti fungal activity of ten essential oils in Vitro. *Microbios* 86: (349) 237 – 245.

Quisumbing, E. 1978. Medicinal plants of the Philippines. Bur.Print., Manila , 1234p.

Shivpuri, A., Sharma, O.P. and Jhamaria, S.L. 1997, Fungitoxic properties of Plant extracts against pathogenic fungi., *Journal of Mycology and Plant pathology.* 27 (1) April ,29 – 31.

Summerfield, A., Keil, G.M., Mettenteitee, T.C., Rzhia, H.J. and Saalmuller, A. 1997. Anti viral activity of an extract from leaves of the tropical plant *Acanthospermum hispidum. Anti viral Research* 36: 55-62.

Tandan, S.K., Chandra, S., Tripathi, H.C. and Lal, J. 1994. Pharmacological effects of *Ageratum conyzoidoes* roots. *Indian – Journal of Pharmaceutical Sciences* 56: 5, 182 –1 84; 10 ref.

Udupa, A.K., Kulkarni, D.R. and Udupa, S.L. 1995. Effect of *Tridax Procumbens* extracts on wound healing. *International Journal of Parmacognosy*., 33: 37-40. 2 ref.

Varier, P.S.V. 1994, 95 and 96, *Indian Medicinal Plants*, Orient Longman Hyderabad, Volume 1, 2, 3,4 and 5.

Vera, R. 1993. Chemical composition of the essential oil *Ageratum conyzoides* L. (Asteraceae) from Reunion. *Flavour and Fragrance Journal* , 8: 5, 257-260, 24 ref.

Wandji, J., Bissangoa, M.F., Ouambra, J.M., Silou, T., Abena, A.A. and Keita, A. 1996. The essential oil of *Ageratum conyzoides* (French) Fitoterapia 67 (5). 427-431.

Wealth of India 1948-1976. A dictionary of Indian raw materials. Raw material series. Vols. I-III, VI, XI Council of Scientific and Industrial Research, New Delhi.

Zollo, A.P.H. et al. 1995. The Occurrence of 1-Phenyl hepta-1, 3, 5-triyne in the Essential Oil of *Bidens pilosa* L. from Cameroon. *Flavour Fragr. J.*, Vol. 10, 97-100.

Glossary of Medical Terms

1. Abortifacient—A drug that induces abortion
2. Albuminuria—Proteinuria, the presence of serum albumin or other serum proteins in the urine.
3. Alexeteric—Protective to infectious diseases
4. Alexipharmic—A drug used to neutralise a poison; antidote; antipharmic.
5. Alopecia—Loss of hair–a malady in which the hair falls from one or more circumscribed round or oval areas, leaving the skin smooth and white
6. Amenorrhoea—The absence or stopping of menstrual periods.
7. Amentia—Failure of development of the intellectual faculties.
8. Amnesia—Total or partial loss of memory following physical injury, disease drugs or psychological trauma.
9. Anaemia—Reduction in the quantity of the oxygen carrying pigment hoemoglobin in the blood.
10. Analgesic—A drug that relieves pain.
11. Anasarca—Massive swelling of the legs, trunk and genitalia due to retention of fluid found in congestive heart failure and some forms of renal failure.

12. Angina pectoris—Pain in the center of chest, induced by exercise.
13. Anodyne—Any treatment or drug that soothes and eases pain.
14. Anorexia—Loss of appetite.
15. Anthelmintic—Any drug used to destroy parasitic worms.
16. Antibacterial—Directed or effective against bacteria.
17. Anticonvulsant—A drug that reduces or prevent the severity of fits in various types of epilepsy.
18. Antiperiodic—Preventing the regular recurrence of a diseases
19. Antipyretic—A drug that reduces fever by lowering the body temperature.
20. Antispasmodic—A drug that relieves spasm of smooth muscle.
21. Aphrodisiac—An agent that stimulates sexual excitement.
22. Appetiser—An agent that stimulates appetite.
23. Ascariasis—A disease caused by an infestation with the parasitic worm Ascarfs *lumbricoides.*
24. Ascites—The accumulation of fluid in the peritoneal cavity causing abdominal swelling.
25. Asphyxia—Suffocation.
26. Asthma—A condition characterised by paroxysmal attacks of bronchospasm causing difficulty in breathing.
27. Astringent—A drug that causes cells to shrink by precipitating proteins from their surfaces.
28. Biliousness—Affected by the disorder of bile.
29. Blepharitis—inflammations of the eyelids.
30. Bronchitis—Inflammation of the bronchi.
31. Carminative—A drug that relieves flatulence.
32. Cataract—Any opacity of the lens of the eye.
33. Catarrh—The excessive secretion of thick phlegm or mucus by mucus membrane of the nose, nasal sinuses etc.

34. Cephalalgia—Headache
35. Cervicitis—Inflammations of the neck (cervix) of the womb.
36. Cholera—An acute infection of the small intestine by the bacterium *vibrio cholerae* which causes severe vomiting and diarrhoea leading to dehydration.
37. Colic—Severe abdominal pain.
38. Conjunctivitis—Inflammation of the conjunctiva.
39. Constipation—A condition in which bowel evacuations occur infrequently or in which the faeces are hard, and passage causes difficulty or pain.
40. Convulsion—An involuntary contraction of the muscles producing contortion of the body and limbs.
41. Cramp—Prolonged painful contraction of a muscle.
42. Cutaneous diseases—Diseases relating to the skin.
43. Cytotoxic—Damages or destroys cells.
44. Deobstruent—A drug that removes functional obstructions of the body.
45. Dermatitis—Inflammation of the skin caused by an outside agent.
46. Diabetes—Any disorder of carbohydrate metabolism.
47. Diaphoretic—A drug that causes an increase in sweating.
48. Diarrhoea—A common symptom of gastrointestinal diseases resulting in frequent discharge of watery stools.
49. Diuretic—A drug that increases the volume of urine produced by promoting the excretion of salts and water from the kidney.
50. Dropsy—Excessive accumulation of fluid in the body tissues.
51. Dysentery—An infection of the intestinal tract causing severe diarrhoea with blood and mucus.
52. Dysmenorrhoea—Painful or difficult menstruation.
53. Dysopia—Defective vision
54. Dyspepsia—Indigestion or disordered digestion.

55. Dysuria—Difficulty or pain while passing urine.
56. Eczema—A superficial inflammation of the skin, mainly affecting the epidermis.
57. Elephantiasis—Gross enlargement of the skin and underlying connective tissues caused by obstruction of lymph vessels.
58. Embrocat—To moisten and rub
59. Emetic —Causing vomiting
60. Emmenagogue—An agent that stimulates menstruation.
61. Emollient–Softening.
62. Epilepsy—Any one of a group of disorders of brain function characterized by recurrent attacks that have a sudden onset.
63. Epistaxis—Bleeding from the nose which may be caused by physical injury, fever, blood pressure or blood disorders.
64. Erythema—Abnormal flushing of the skin caused by dilation of the blood capillaries.
65. Expectorant—A drug that enhances the secretion of sputum by the air passage.
66. Febrifuge—A drug that prevents fever.
67. Fit–A sudden attack, this term is usually reserved for the attacks of epilepsy.
68. Flatulence—The expulsion of gas or air from stomach through the mouth.
69. Galactagogue–Medicine that promotes secretion of milk
70. Galactogogue—An agent that stimulates the secretion of milk.
71. Gastropathy–Any disease of the stomach
72. Giddiness—Tending to fall or stagger.
73. Gonorrhoea—A venereal disease caused by the bacterium *Neisseria gonorrhoeas* that affects the genital mucous of membrane of either sex.
74. Gout—A disease in which a defect in uric acid metabolism causes an excess of the acid and its salts to accumulate in the blood stream and joints.
75. Gravel—Small stones formed in the urinary tract.

76. Haematomesi—Morbid state due to infestation with worms.
77. Haematuria—The presence of blood in the urine.
78. Haemoptysis—The coughing up of blood.
79. Haemorrhoid—A bleeding pile
80. Haemorrhoids—Enlarged veins in the walls of anus (Piles).
81. Haemostatic—Styptic.
82. Haemostatic—An agent that stops or prevents hoemorrhage.
83. Helminthiasis—The diseased condition resulting from an infestation with parasitic worms.
84. Hepatitis—Inflammation of the liver; jaundice
85. Hepatopathy—Any disease of the liver.
86. Hiccough—Abrupt involuntary lowering of diaphragm and closure of the sound producing folds at the upper end of the trachea, producing a characteristic sound as the breath is drawn in.
87. Hydrophobia—An acute virus disease of the central nervous system that affects mammals and is usually transmitted to man by a bite from an infected dog.
88. Hypnotic—A drug that produces sleep by depressing brain function.
89. Hysteria—A neurosis whose principal features consists of emotional instability, repression etc.
90. Icterus—Jaundice.
91. Indigestion—Disordered digestion.
92. Inflammation—The immediate defensive reaction of tissue to any injury, which may be caused by infection, chemicals or physical agents.
93. Insanity—A degree of mental illness.
94. Insomnia—Inability to fall asleep.
95. Lactagogue—An agent that stimulates secretion of milk.
96. Larvicidal—An agent that kills larva.

97. Laxative—A drug used to stimulate or increase the frequency of bowel evacuation or to encourage a softer or bulkier stool.
98. Leprosy—A chronic disease caused by *Mycobacterium leprae,* that affects the skin, mucous membranes and nerves.
99. Leucoderma—A skin condition characterized by defective whitish pigmentation; a congenital absence of pigments in spot.
100. Leucorrhoea—A whitish or yellowish discharge of mucus from the vaginal opening.
101. Lithotripsy—An agent thought to be effective in dissolving various concretions in the body.
102. Malaria—An infectious disease due to the presence of parasitic protozoa.
103. Menorrhagia – Excessive or prolonged menstruation.
104. Myopia—Short sightedness.
105. Nausea—The feeling that one is about to vomit.
106. Necrotic—Dead or dying, especially in reference to tissues of a certain area.
107. Neuralgic—A severe burning or stabbing pain often following the course of a nerve.
108. Obesity—The condition in which excess fat has accumulated in the body.
109. Odontalgia—Toothache.
110. Ophthalmopathy – Any disease of the eye.
111. Ophthamia—A term usually applied to conjunctivitis.
112. Otalgia—Pain in the ear.
113. Pectoral—Effective on diseases of the chest.
114. Pertusis—Whooping cough.
115. Pharyngitis—Inflammation of the part of the throat behind the soft palate.
116. Pharyngodynia—Pain in the pharynx
117. Pharyngopathy—Diseases of pharynx.

118. Plague—An epidemic disease with a high death rate transmitted by rat fleas.
119. Pneumonia—Inflammation of the lung caused by viruses or unknown agents.
120. Pruritis—Itching.
121. Psoriasis—A chronic skin diseases in which itchy scaly red patches form on the elbows, for arms, knees, legs etc.
122. Purgative—Laxative.
123. Refrigerant—Reducing thirst or having a cooling effect on the surface of the body.
124. Rheumatism—Any disorder in which aches and pains affect the muscles and joints.
125. Scabies— A skin infection caused by the itch mite, *Sarcoptes scabiei.*
126. Sedative—A drug that has a calming effect, relieving anxiety and tension.
127. Smallpox—An acute infectious virus disease causing high fever and a rash that scars the skin.
128. Sore throat—Pain at the back of the mouth.
129. Spasmodic—Occurring in spasms.
130. Stimulant—An agent that promotes the activity of a body system or function.
131. Stomachalgia—Pain in the stomach.
132. Stomachic—An agent that stimulates the secretory activity of the stomach.
133. Styptic–Having the power to arrest bleeding
134. Syphilis—Chronic venereal disease caused by the bacterium *Treponema pallidum,* resulting in the formation of lesions throughout the body.
135. Tetanus—An acute infectious disease affecting th nervous system.
136. Tremor—A rhythmical alternating movement that may affect any part of the body.

137. Tuberculosis—An infectious disease caused by the bacillus *Mycobacterium tuberculosis.*

138. Ulcer—A break in the skin or in the mucous membrane lining the alimentary tract that fails to heal and is often accompanied by inflammation.

139. Vermifuge—Any drug or chemical agent used to expel worms from the intestine.

140. Vesical – Anatomy & Medicine relating to or affecting the urinary bladder

141. Vitilago—Leucoderma

142. Whooping cough—An acute contagious disease, primarily affecting children, due to infection of the mucous membranes lining the air passage.

Gas chromatograms of various essential oil yielding plants of Asteraceae

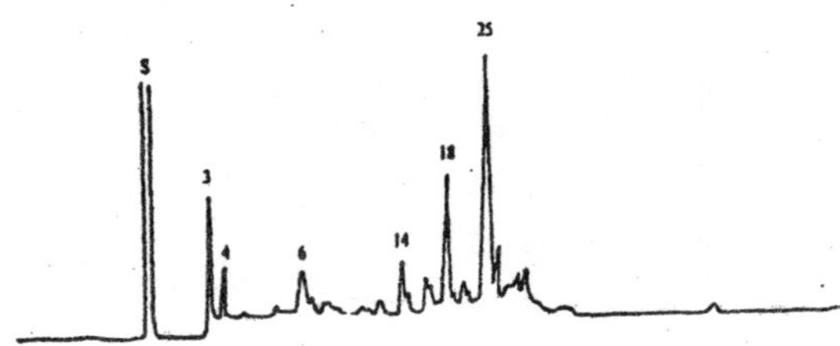

Chromolaena odorata (Eupatorium odoratum) (7e)

S – Solvent, 3 – alpha-Pinene, 4 – beta-Pinene, 6 – Limonene, 14 – Thymol, 18 – Carvacrol, 25 – beta-Caryophyllene

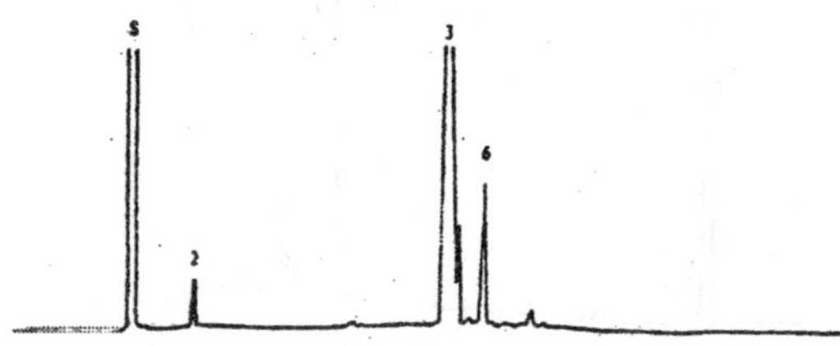

Eupatoprium triplinerve (8e)

S – Solvent, 2 – alpha-Pinene, 3 – Cravacrol, 6 – beta-Caryophyllene

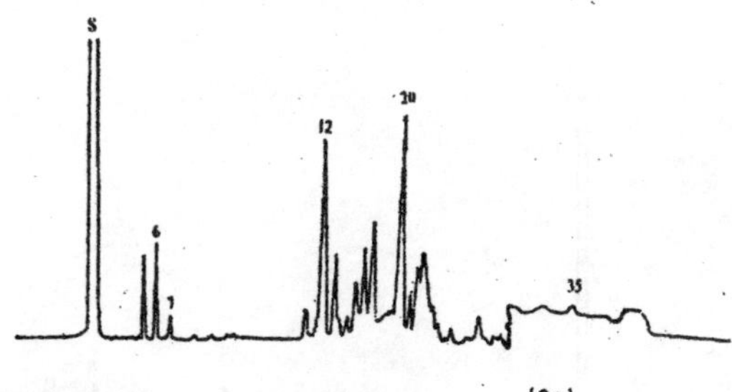

Mikania cordata (9e)

S – Solvent, 6 – alpha-Pinene, 7 – beta-Pinene, 12 – Thymol, 20 – beta-Caryophyllene, 35 – Germacrene-D

Gas chromatograms of various essential oil yielding plants of Asteraceae

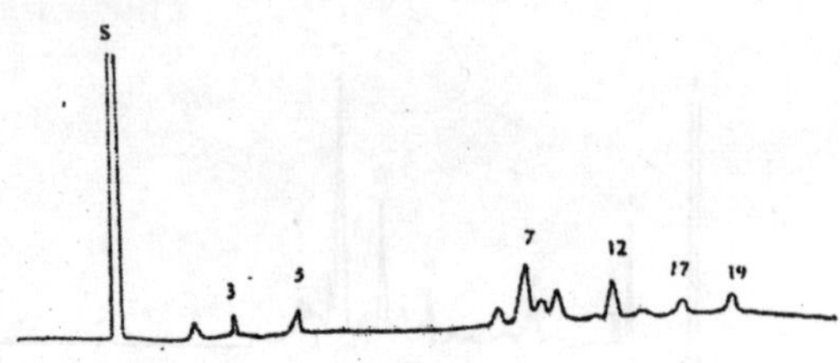

(3e)

Vernonia cinerea

S – Solvent, 3 – Linalool, 5 – Terpenen-4-ol, 7 – beta-Caryophyllene, 12 – Humulene, 17 – Germacrene-D, 19 – delta-Cadinene

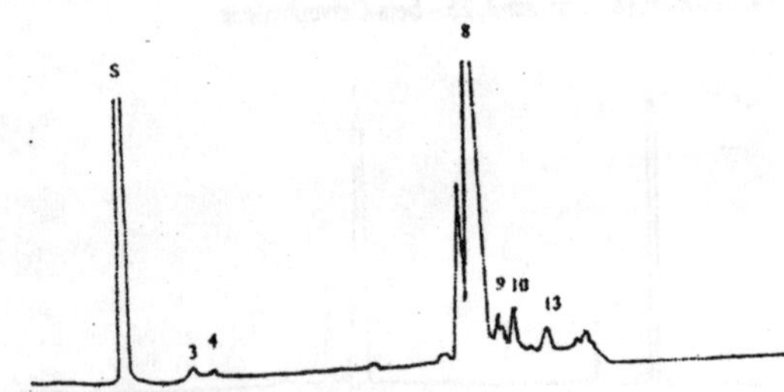

(5e)

Ageratum conyzoides

S – Solvent, 3 – alpha-Pinene, 4 – Phellandrene, 8 – Unidentified, 9 – beta-Elemene, 10 – beta-Bisabolene, 13 – beta-Caryophyllene

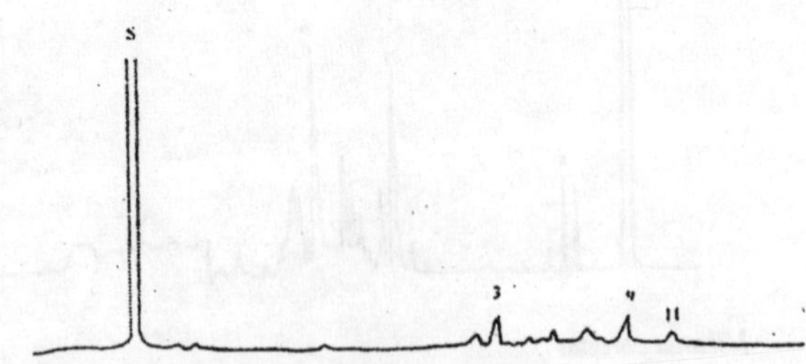

(6e)

Ageratum houstonianum

S – Solvent, 3 – alpha-Farnesene, 9 – Germacrene-D, 11 – delta-Cadinene

Gas chromatograms of various essential oil yielding plants of Asteraceae

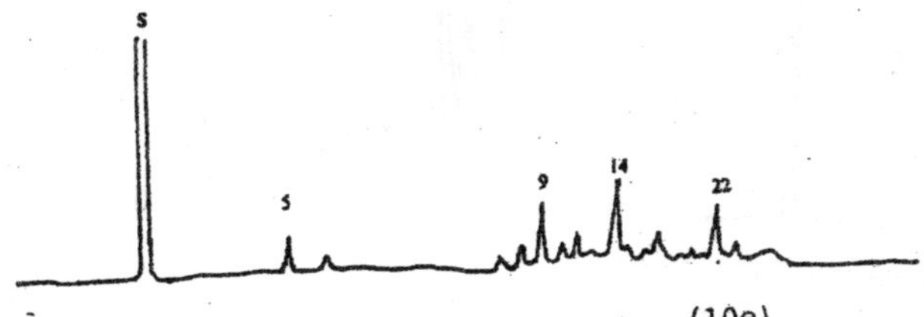

Conyza bonariensis
S – Solvent, 5 – Limonene, 9 – beta-Caryophyllene, 14 – Humulene, 22 – Farnesene

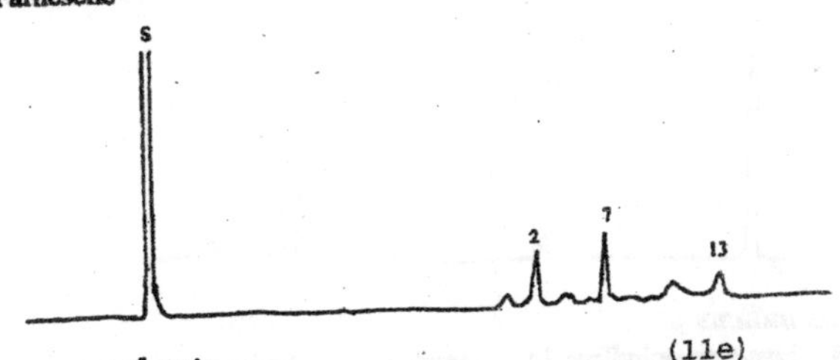

Conyza canadensis
S – Solvent, 2 – beta-Cayophyllene, 7 – Humulene, 13 – delta-Cadinene

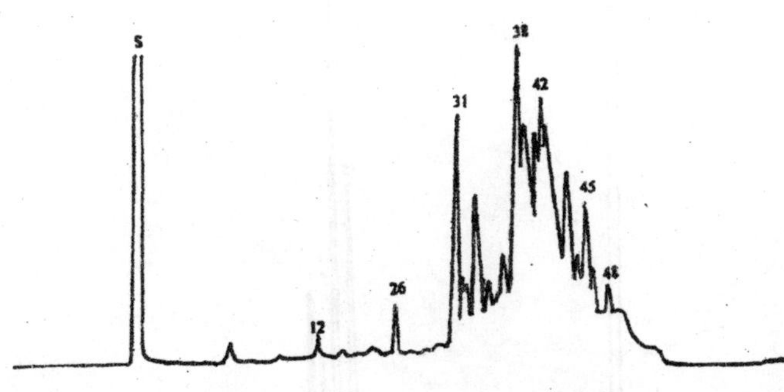

Blumea lacera
S – Solvent, 12 – Terpenen-4-ol, 26 – Eugenol, 31 – beta-Caryophyllene, 38 – Humulene, 42 – Selinene, 45 – Germacrene-D, 48 - delta-Cadinene

Gas chromatograms of various essential oil vielding plants of Asteraceae

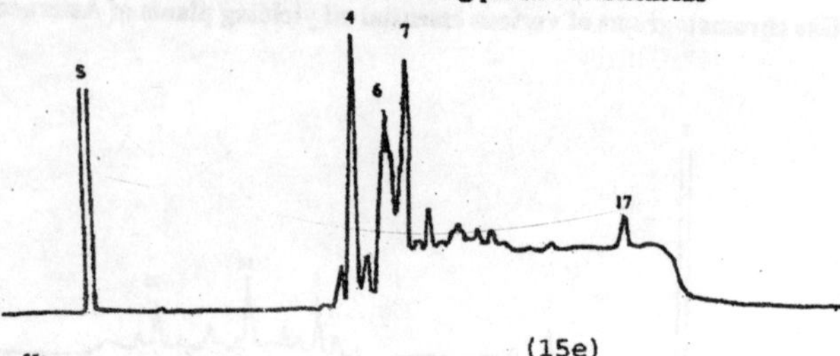

Blumea mollis

S – Solvent, 4 – Linalyl acetate, 6 – beta-Bisabolene, 7 – beta-Caryophyllene, 17 – delta-Cadinene

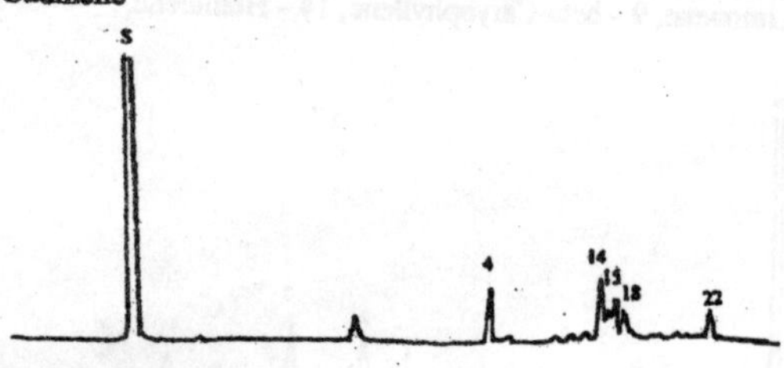

Sphaeranthus indicus (17e)

S – Solvent, 4 – beta-Caryophyllene, 14 – Humulene, 15 – Selinene, 18 – Ionone, 22 – delta-Cadinene

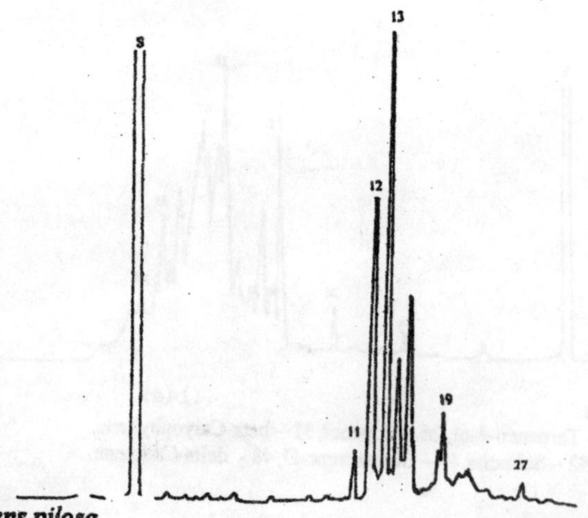

Bidens pilosa (20e)

S – Solvent, 11 – beta Elemene, 12 – beta Bisabolene, 13 – beta- Caryophyllene, 19 – Humulene, 27 - Germacrene-D

Gas chromatograms of various essential oil yielding plants of Asteraceae

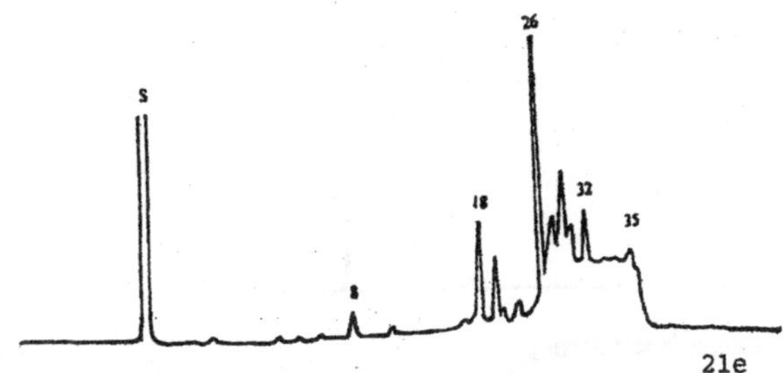

21e

Cosmos bipinntus cv. orange
S – Solvent, 8 – Terpenen-4-ol, 18 – beta-Caryophyllene, 26 – Humulen
32 – Germacrene-D, 35 – delta-Cadinene

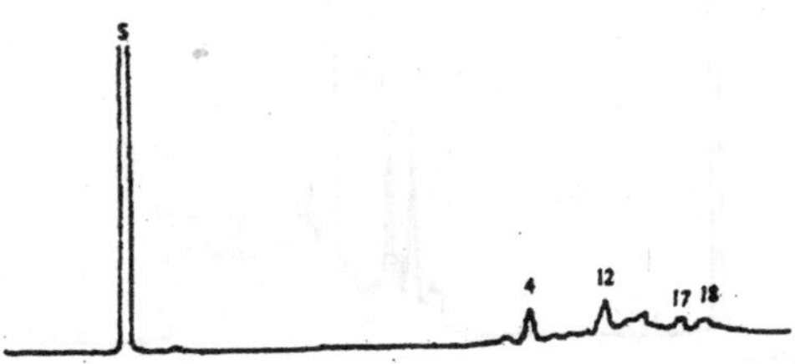

22e

Cosmos bipinnatus cv. yellow
S – Solvent, 4 – beta-Caryophyllene, 12 – Humulene, 17 – Germacrene-D,
18 – delta-Cadinene

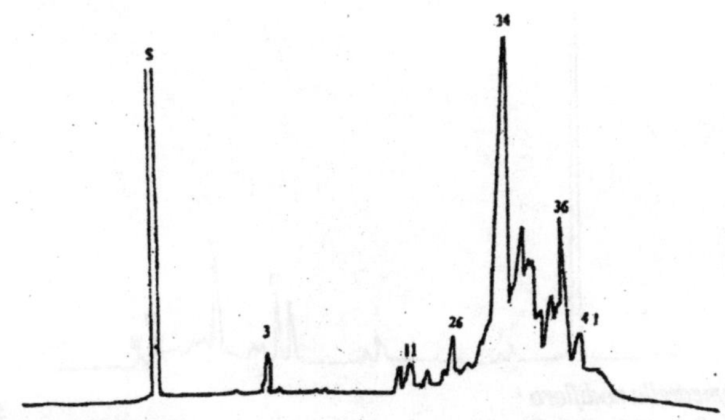

Cosmos caudatus

23e

S – Solvent, 3 – Limonene, 11 – Linalyl acetate, 26 – beta-Caryophyllene,
34 – Humulene, 36 – Germacrene-D, 41 – delta-Cadinene

Gas chromatograms of various essential oil yielding plants of Asteraceae

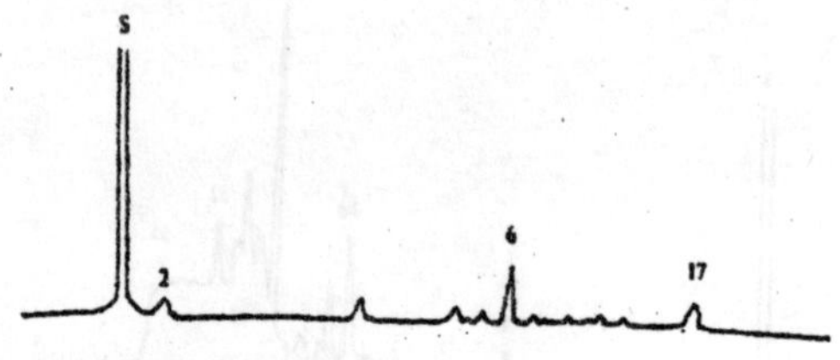

Parthenium hysterophor us 27e

S – Solvent, 2 – alpha-Pinene, 6 – beta-Caryophyllene, 17 – Delta-Cadinene

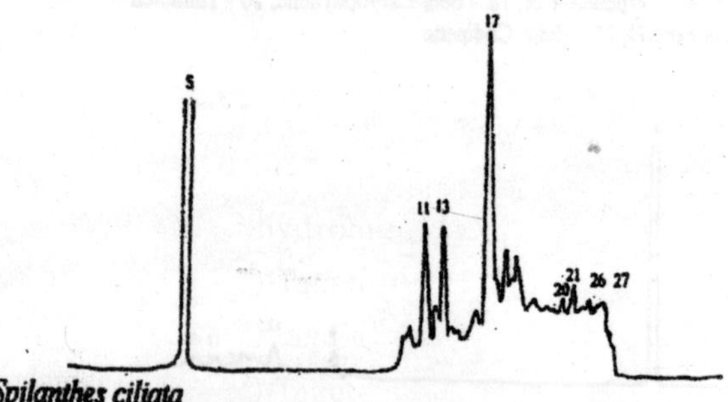

Spilanthes ciliata 30e

S – Solvent, 11 – Thymol, 13 – Methyl chavicol, 17 – beta-Caryophyllene, 20 – Humulene , 21 – beta-Selinene, 26 – Germacrene-D, 27 – delta-Cadinene

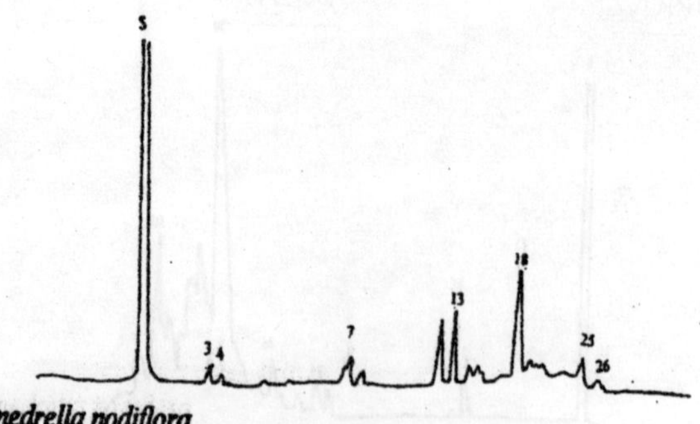

Synedrella nodiflora 33e

S – Solvent, 3 – alpha-Pinene, 4 – beta-Pinene, 7 – Limonene, 13 – beta-Caryophyllene, 18 – Farnesene, 25 – Germacrene-D, 26 – delta-Cadinene

Gas chromatograms of various essential oil yielding plants of Asteraceae

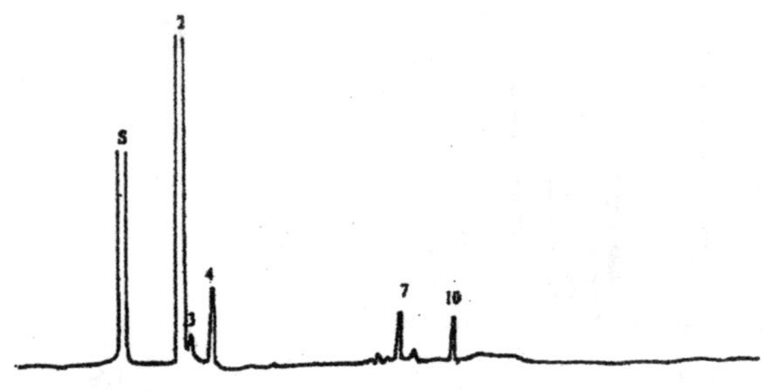

36e

Wedelia chinensis

S – Solvent, 2 – alpha-Pinene, 3 – beta-Pinene, 4– Limonene, 7 – Borneol, 10 – beta-Caryophyllene

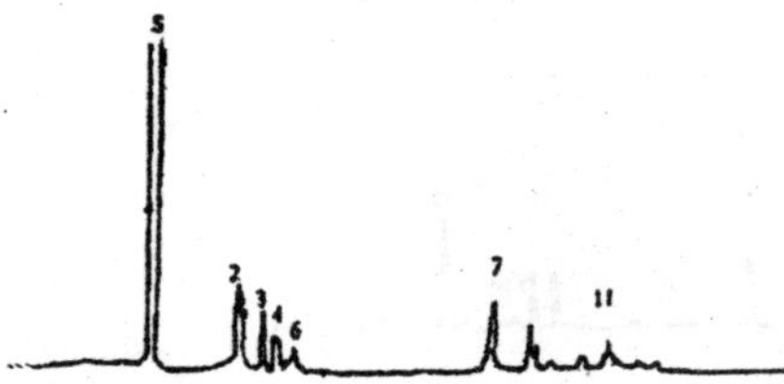

37e

Wedelia trilobata

S – Solvent, 2 – alpha-Pinene, 3 – beta-Pinene, 4 – beta-Phellandrene, 6 – Limonene, 7 – Thymol, 11 – beta-Caryophyllene

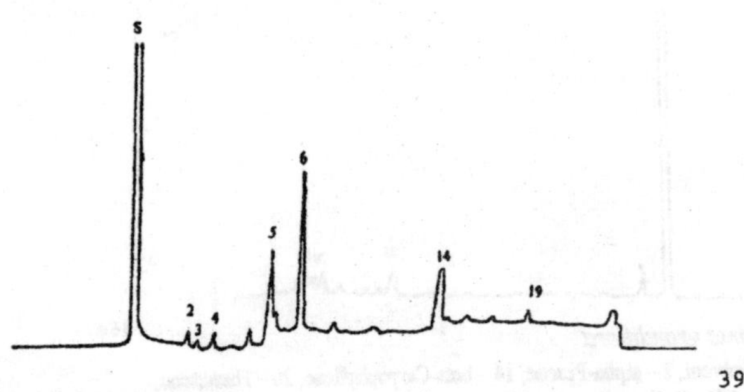

39e

Tagetes erecta c v orange

S – Solvent, 2 - alpha-Pinene, 3 – beta-Pinene, 4 – Sabinene, 5 – Limonene, 6 – Linalool, 14 – beta-Caryophyllene, 19 – Piperitone

Gas chromatograms of various essential oil yielding plants of Asteraceae

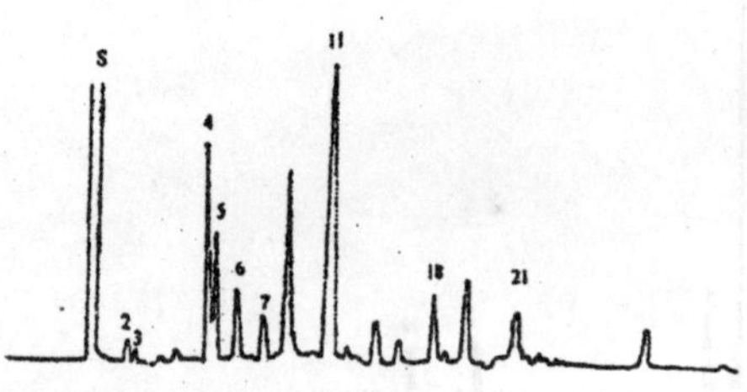

Tagetes patula 42e

S – Solvent, 2 – alpha-Pinene, 3 – beta-Pinene, 4 – Sabinene, 5 – beta-Phellandrene, 6 – Limonene, 7 – Linalool, 11 – Thymol, 18 – beta-Caryophyllene, 21 – Piperitone

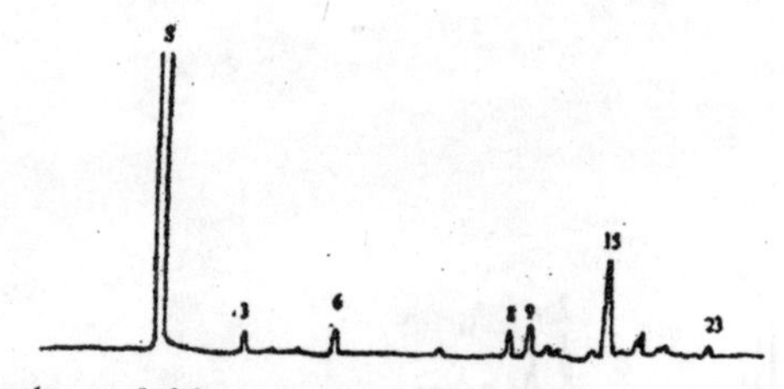

Emilia sonchifolia 45e

S – Solvent, 3 – Linalool, 6 – Terpene-4-ol, 8 – beta-Bisabolene, 9 – beta- Caryophyllene, 15 – Humulene, 23 – Germacrene-D

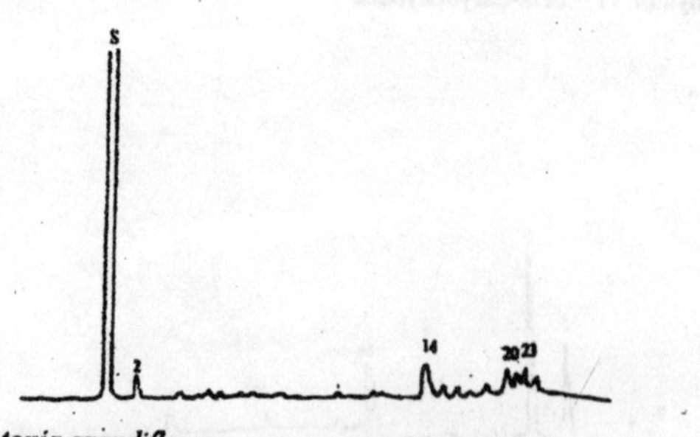

Notonia grandiflora 46e

S – Solvent, 2 – alpha-Pinene, 14 – beta-Caryophyllene, 20 – Humulene, 23 – delta-Cadinene

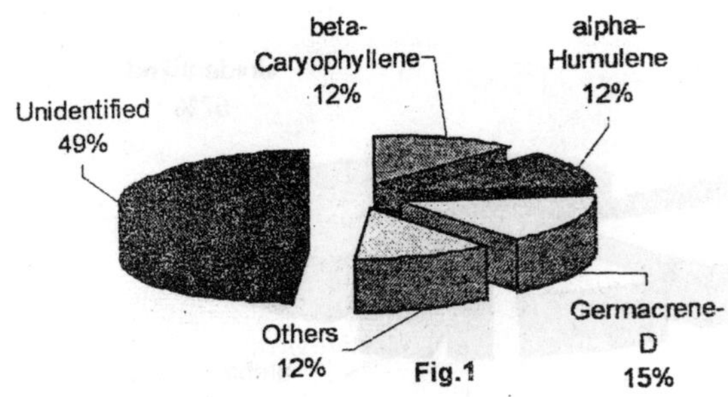

Fig.1

Vernonia cinerea

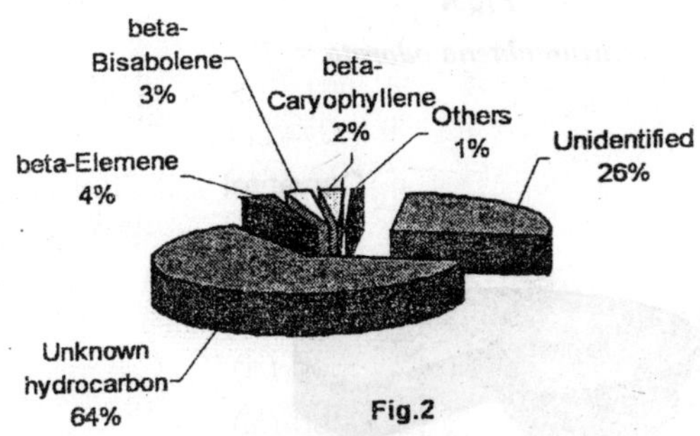

Fig.2

Ageratum conyzoides

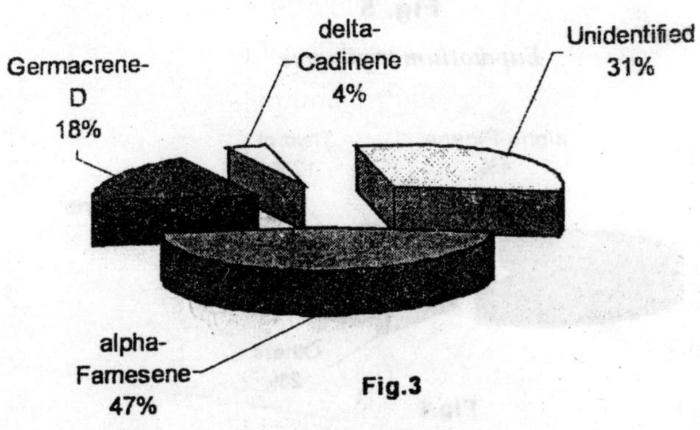

Fig.3

Ageratum haustonianum

Others
3%
Unidentified
57%
beta-
Caryophyllene
21%
Carvacrol
11%
Thymol
3%
alpha-Pinene
5%

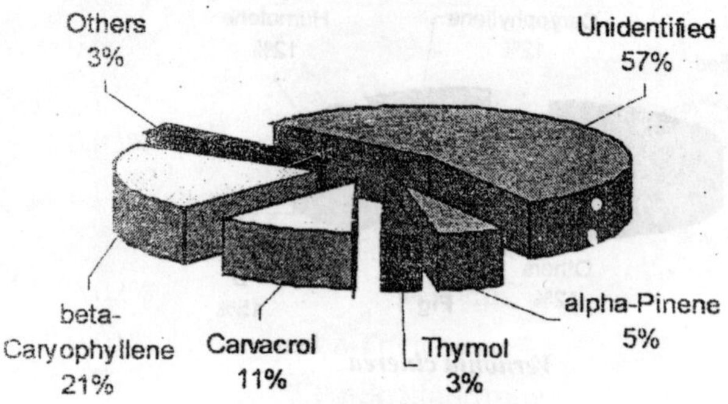

Fig.4

Chromolaena odorata

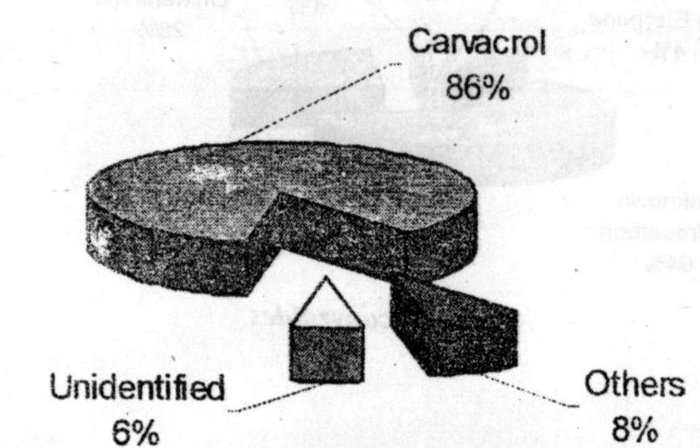

Fig. 5

Eupatorium triplinerve

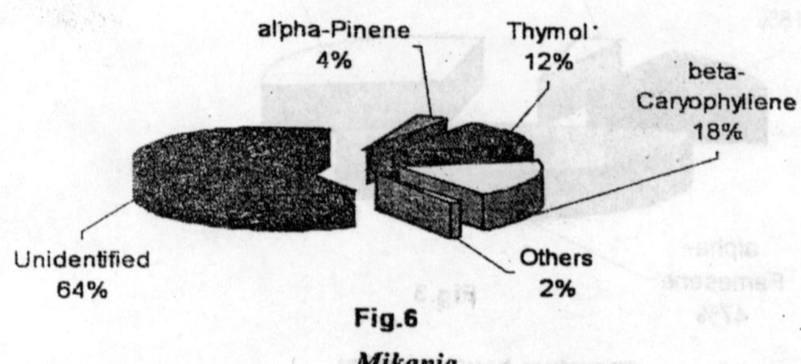

Fig.6

Mikania

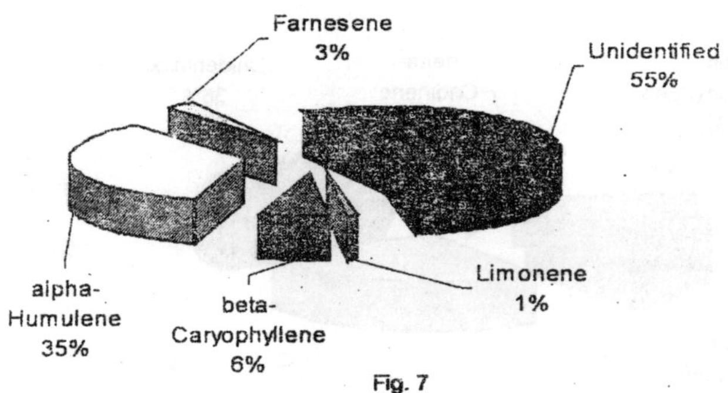

Fig. 7

Conyza bonariensis

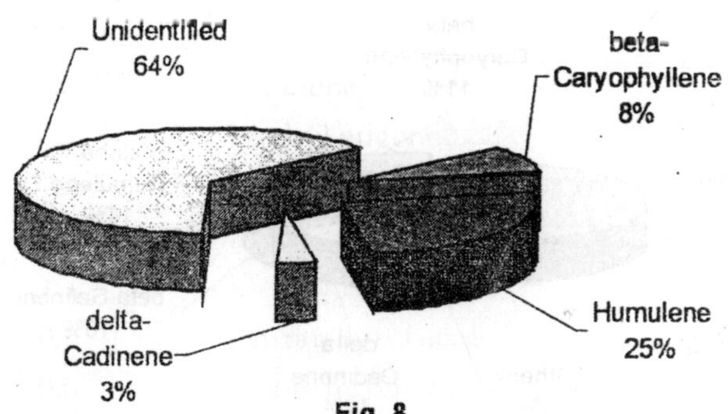

Fig. 8

Conyza canadensis

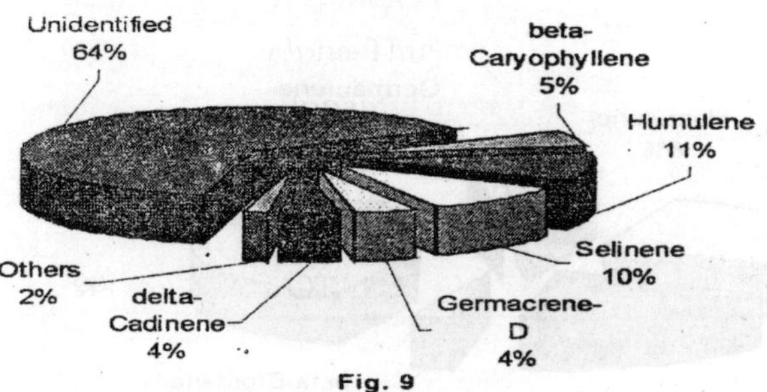

Fig. 9

Blumea lacera

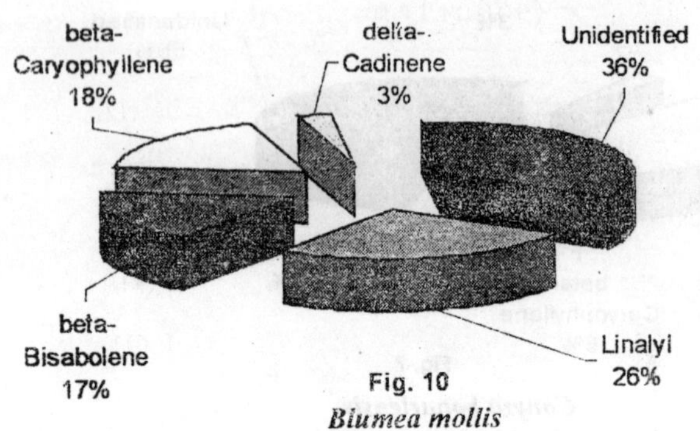

Fig. 10

Blumea mollis

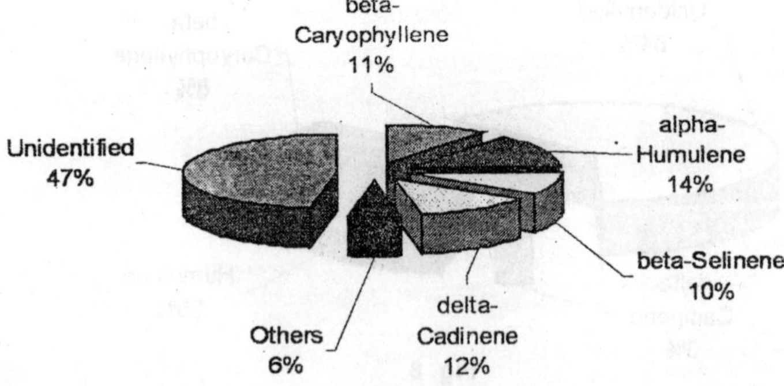

Fig. 11

Sphaeranthus indicus

beta-
Caryophyllen
e
27%
Humulene
6%
Germacrene-
D
1%
Unidentified
43%
beta-
Bisabolene
20%
beta-Elemene
3%

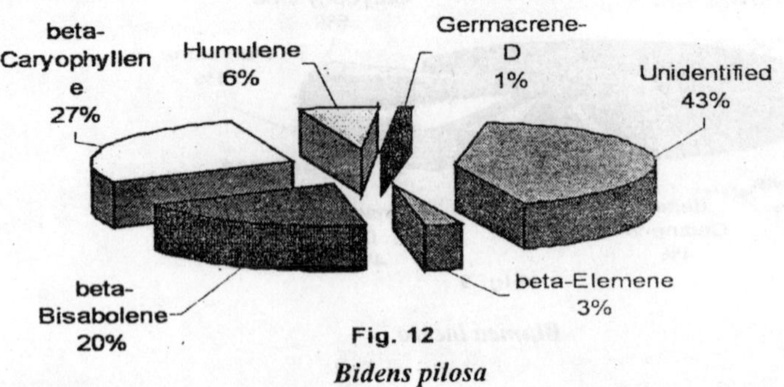

Fig. 12

Bidens pilosa

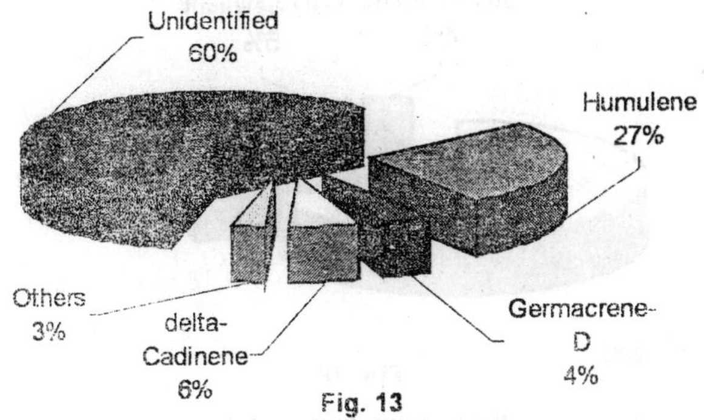

Fig. 13

Cosmos bipinnatus cv orange

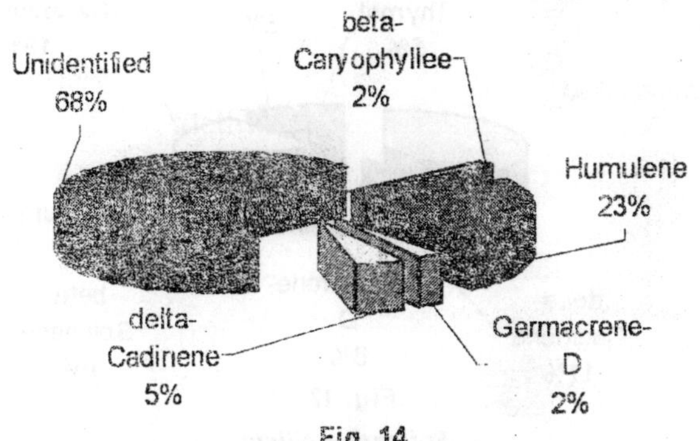

Fig. 14

Cosmos bipinnatus cv yellow

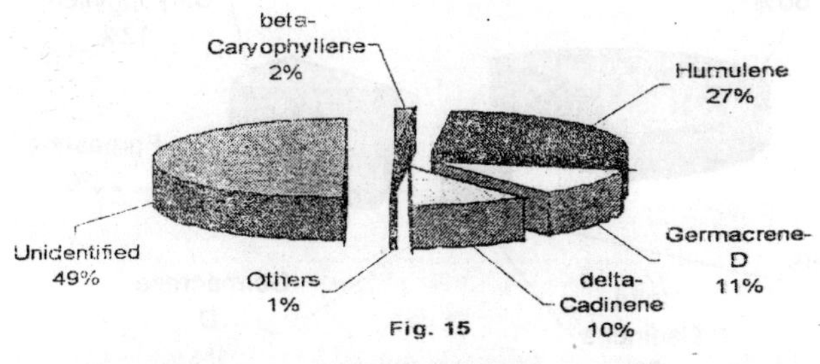

Fig. 15

Cosmos caudatus

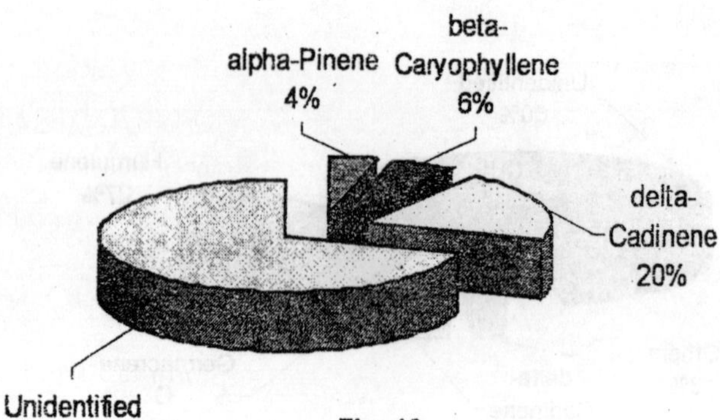

Fig. 16

Parthenium hysterophorus

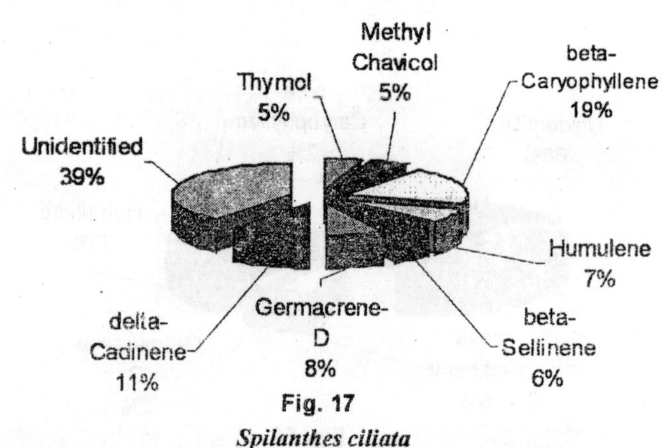

Fig. 17

Spilanthes ciliata

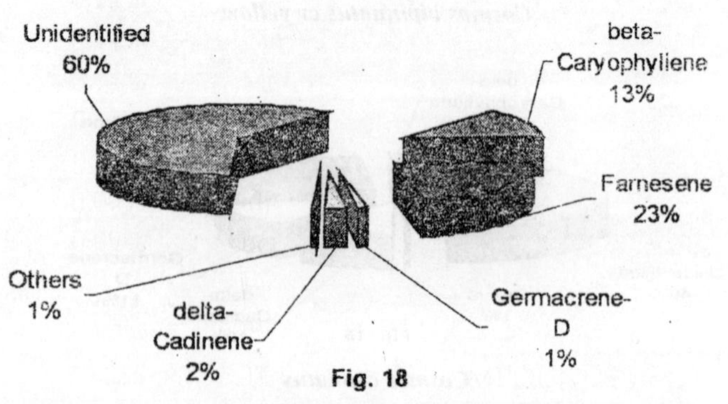

Fig. 18

Synedrella nodiflora

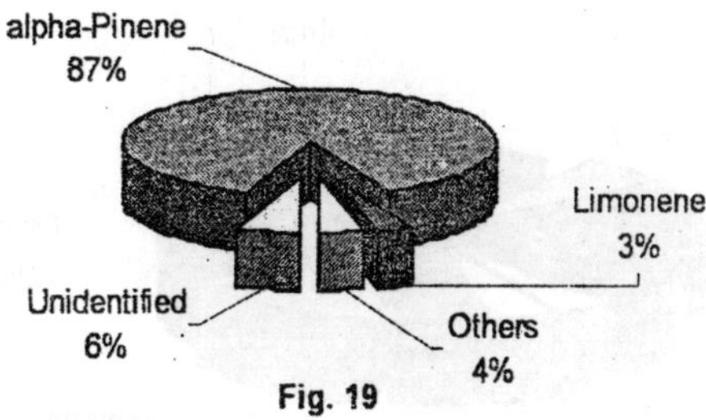

Fig. 19

Wedelia chinensis

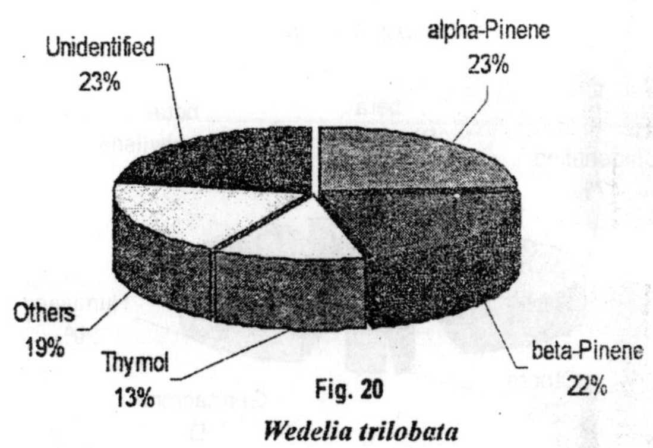

Fig. 20

Wedelia trilobata

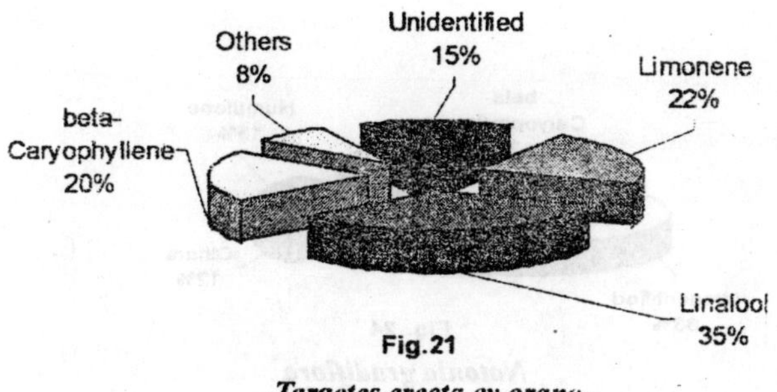

Fig.21

Targetes erecta cv orang

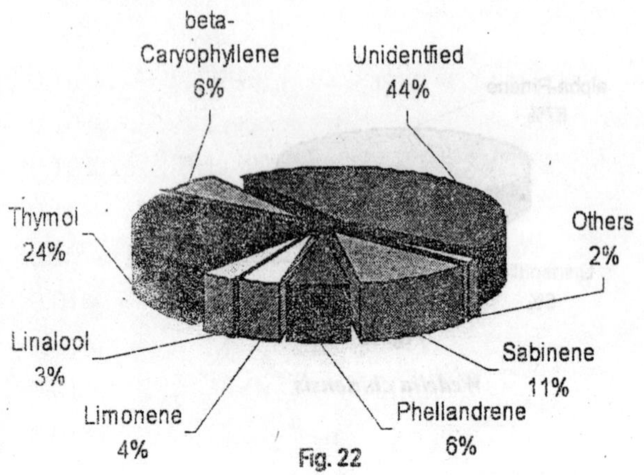

Fig. 22

Targetes patula

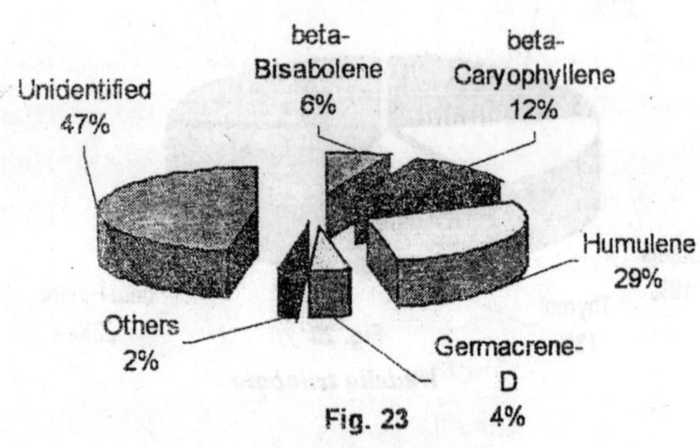

Fig. 23

Emilia sonchifolia

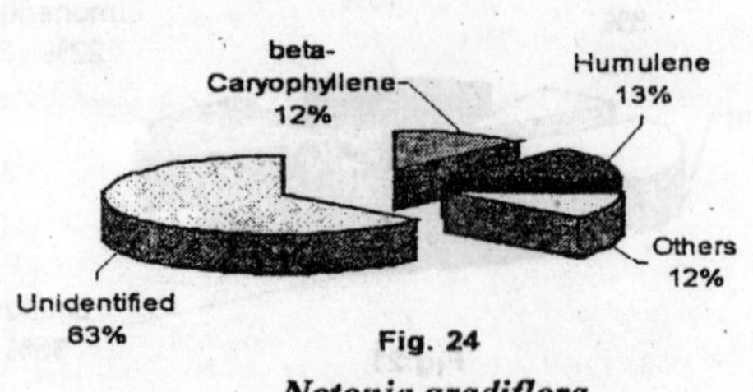

Fig. 24

Notonia gradiflora